T0107191

Tantric Sex for Women

ABOUT THE AUTHOR

Christa Schulte, born in 1953, lives with her love- and life-partner in
Bremen, Germany, where she operates her own center for feminist
psychotherapy and supervision. In addition to a degree in Integrative
Gestalt therapy, training in physical therapy, and ten-year training in belly
dancing, she has learned various forms of tantra, and she now mainly
works with women on the issues of self-love and sexuality.

For several years she has been developing her own theories on the cultivation of female sexuality, called Tara-Tantra, concepts upon which this
book is based.

A really inciting and exciting book ... for women of all sexual preferences.... Christa Schulte uses language that is **affectionate, humorous
and enchanting.**... *Tantric Sex for Women* is more than a guide to more
fulfilling sex for individual women. I hope this book will initiate a
discussion that fundamentally questions some of the widespread convic-
tions about female sexuality.... If we have the courage to transcend the
prohibitions and taboos that we have taken over from our childhood, not
just relationships among women but also those between women and men
will improve significantly.
— Marianne Krüll, *ab 40*, 2001

Humorous, knowledgeable and self-confident, she offers food for
thought and practical advice for women who want to cultivate their sexuality and sensuality....
— *Querelle 9*, 2001

Tantric Sex for Women, the **highly praised** book by Christa Schulte, offers a
variety of tips for everyday ecstasies and special occasions....
— *Queer.de*, July 2001

Another Tantra-book? Yes, but one that starts with the **singularity of
female sexuality.**
— *KGS Bremen (Körper, Geist, Seele = Body, Mind, Spirit)*

Christa Schulte wants to cultivate pleasure. It's about sex and much
more: it's about the connection "to the heart," about meditation, and
about dignity. "We live in an ecstasy-phobic society," says Schulte.
"There are sexualized images en masse, but they don't really ignite sexual
energy, at least not in women." That's exactly the task that this Tantra
teacher has set for herself. For women only. [...] "For many, it is healing
to be able to show their pleasure with dignity, and with pride in their
bodies, in the presence of another.... Fears are there to be overcome."
— Susanne Gieffers, *taz Bremen*, 15/16 December 2001

Tantric Sex
FOR *Women*

A GUIDE FOR LESBIAN, BI, HETERO AND SOLO LOVERS

Christa Schulte

Translated from the German by Emily Banwell

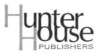

LIBRARY OF CONGRESS CATALOGING-IN-PUBLICATION DATA
Schulte, Christa.
    [Tantra für Geniesserinnen. English]
    Tantric sex for women : a guide for lesbian, bi, hetero, and solo lovers / Christa
Schulte.
            p. cm.
    Translation of: Tantra für Geniesserinnen.
    Includes bibliographical references and index.
    ISBN-13: 978-0-89793-445-9 (pbk.)
    ISBN-10: 0-89793-445-8 (pbk.)
    1. Sex instruction for women. 2. Sex. 3. Tantrism. I. Title.
HQ46.S38 2004
613.9'6—dc22   2004016123

PROJECT CREDITS
Cover Design: Brian Dittmar Graphic Design   Book Production: Hunter House
Photographs (pp. 16, 137, 189): Christiane Pausch, Berlin
Line Illlustrations: Eva Wagendristel (pp. 31, 43); Eric Venuto (p. 27)
Chapter Opener Illustrations: research, Antonia Lee; rendering, Stefanie Gold
Translator: Emily Banwell; Translation Assistance, Elisabeth Wohofsky
Developmental and Copy Editor: Kelley Blewster
Proofreader: John David Marion   Indexers: Robert and Cynthia Swanson
Acquisitions Editor: Jeanne Brondino
Editor: Alexandra Mummery
Publishing Assistant: Antonia T. Lee
Publicist: Jillian Steinberger
Foreign Rights Coordinator: Elisabeth Wohofsky
Customer Service Manager: Christina Sverdrup
Order Fulfillment: Washul Lakdhon
Administrator: Theresa Nelson   Computer Support: Peter Eichelberger
Publisher: Kiran S. Rana

Printed and Bound by Bang Printing, Brainerd, Minnesota

Manufactured in the United States of America
9 8 7 6 5 4 3   First Edition   09 10 11 12 13

Contents

Important Note

The material in this book is intended to provide a review of information regarding tantric sex techniques. Every effort has been made to provide accurate and dependable information.

However, the publisher, authors, and editors, as well as the professionals quoted in the book, cannot be held responsible for any error, omission, professional disagreement, or outdated material and are not liable for any damage, injury, or other adverse outcome due to the use or application of the information contained in this book.

We believe that the sensuality advice given in this book poses no risk to any healthy person. However, if you have any sexually transmitted diseases, we recommend consulting with your doctor before using this book. If you have questions concerning the information described in this book, consult a qualified professional.

Preface

Love, in its manifold forms, is the only thing that counts. And sex is the
most intimate and powerful way to feel and to express it.

This is a book for women who feel desire, who yearn for more pleasure, who are curious and adventurous. It arises from my love for sexual ecstasy and from the fun I have in creating new, playful games. It is also a result of my being touched by all the women who open themselves to love, happiness, and ecstasy in my courses and in individual and couples therapy.

About me: As a licensed psychologist and psychotherapist I have concentrated for about twenty years on ways to support women in (re)discovering their sexuality, finding their innate forms of expression, and further developing, cultivating, and sharing with others the gentle force of their desire—regardless of whether their sexual orientation is heterosexual, bisexual, lesbian, or solo. *Tantric Sex for Women,* a book of games, exercises, and suggestions, grew from seventeen years of pleasure work in many playshops for women. Tantra circles use it regionally and beyond. In Germany, men who are curious and adventurous have read it, and their girlfriends and wives are pleased with the subtle changes they notice in their partners.

Unlike the German edition, the North American edition does not focus solely on women who love women, but is for all women. The focus of the book is on women because there already exist several shelves of tantra literature that include male desire and describe sexual encounters with men. This book is for women who want to liberate their desire from the prison of norms and rules, and who perhaps already have a notion that enjoyable, satisfying sex increases the appetite for more sex, and more, and more....

Where does this lead? To the self-confident, free, courageous, sensual woman who takes the following poem for her orientation:

The sexual love of women is a rebellious seagull,

Who only with loud (psychosomatic) lamentations

Lets herself be locked in the matte-gilded cage of conformist femininity.

If she shrivels in it long enough, she'll stop crying,

And on the familiar path to the feeding dish she even forgets

That she can actually fly.

She only needs to feel a few rays of fiery-ecstatic sun,

And she will fly towards it with her wild-tender wing beats.

Acknowledgments

I would like to thank so many people who were directly or indirectly involved with this book that I can't mention them all by name.

Naturally, my greatest thanks go to Helga, my dearest, who has accompanied me with all her love for eighteen years now and who continually invents new kinds of pleasure with me; her love has also helped my pleasure in the writing of this book to flow.

Many of the games and exercises are my version of exercises and rituals from SkyDancing, developed by Margot Anand, Eva Szabo, and Aman Schröter; from *Das Tao der Frau* (The Tao of the Woman), by Maitreyi Piontek; and from the Quodoushka of the Cherokee women (American Indian tantra). These female pioneers have significantly influenced my own development.

My thanks to all those from whom I learned to live out my pleasure, especially where learning and teaching were interwoven. This goes not only for my teachers, but also for all the women who were my students, clients, supervisees, colleagues, listeners, and well-meaning critical companions. Among these, I thank especially my assistant and organizer, Maria Kennerknecht, whose ideas and critiques are valuable to me.

Really helping me to stay "on task" were Renate Kösling, Marianne Sörensen, Sangit Kirchner, and several other friends, including Claudia Kroll, who helped with the writing, and Ingelore Hagel, who gave tips and good advice. I also appreciate my Westphalian grandma, from whom I inherited my own combination of a love of pleasure and discipline, which gave me the ability to finish this book.

✻ FOR HELGA ✻

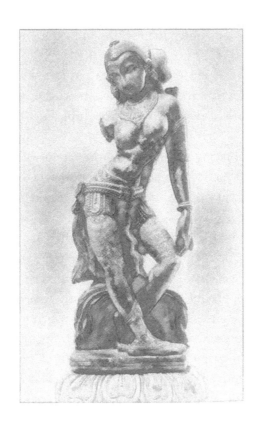

Introduction

*S*ex is one way to experience and express love, passion, tenderness, sensuality, and intimacy.

Sex is also one way for adult women to play, to experience others physically, and to encounter themselves and others with closeness and pleasure.

Sex, as one way of expressing pleasure and love, can be cultivated and refined to become a true *art* through love, knowledge, will, talent (accompanied with self-love), and above all through playing, experimenting, and practicing.

The ideas of playing and experimenting are usually preferred to the idea of practice. Practice is associated—wrongly, I believe—with performance pressure, physical education, and boring repetitions. When we see a ballet dancer float across the stage like a fairy, we know—however moved we may be by her body's expression—that she trains hard at least eight hours a day and that she has her tense muscles massaged afterward. Her skill, then, is seen as an art.

Loving, lustful, playful, creative, and possibly even spiritual sexuality is also an art, and it comes (besides from talent, which we will ignore here) from a desire for love and self-expression, from trying out, from practicing, and finally from knowing how. And this is without any need for "hard" training! But how can an orgasm (in which, after all, a few highly physical parts play a role, in addition to the mind and spirit) find its depth and length when your pelvic muscles are still in a deep sleep?

When it comes to sex, women tend to ignore the physical practice aspect because they feel "as long as there is love, it will work out fine." This view often hides an alienated relationship to one's own body and the belief that the other will know, without words, what one needs, and it is based on the idea that an orgasm depends on the love and dexterity of the other. But what about sexual self-love? Or new sexual encounters? And what is female sexuality anyway?

Here's my current subjective definition of female sexuality: *Female sexuality is the totality of that which women imagine to be sexuality, even if they only feel and experience a fragment of it.*

And below are examples of what that might mean, a list of some of the poles between which the pendulum of sexual energy can swing:

Female sexuality is...

Tingling arousal and creeping listlessness

Untamable desire and sudden repulsion

Infinite loss of control and perfectly controlled power play

Sweet arousal and dedicated lethargy

Loving encounter and orgasmic self-centeredness

Cautious tenderness and wild floor acrobatics

Playful eroticism and bold grabbing

High tension in a self-aware border experience and cosmic melting
with the world

Chuckling joy and nameless pain

Many small deaths and newborn life

With these examples of polarized phenomena, I do not want to postulate oppositions where none exist; rather, I want to show ranges of possible pendulum movements. When we consider how many personal life stories, how many established encounter and relationship structures, how many different situations and contexts can give these descriptions their unmistakable character, it becomes clear once again how necessary subjective definitions are for women to properly describe themselves. These definitions are important also for debunking the so-called "objective" definitions formed by the male gaze on female sexuality, which will always be a foreign gaze.

Let's have the courage to allow an inside view, to get insights into the multiplicity of female sexual desire! Let's store all value judgments and verdicts in the fridge of shoulds and mustn'ts, and let us melt with devotion in the heat of sexual ecstasies.

What thereby develops—both spontaneously and with planning—are living art pieces of pleasure. The art of love can be learned, and practicing to get there can be fun! I can only give tips and suggestions for the practical steps toward cultivating the art of love; women know most of this art themselves anyway. If anything, they need the permission (from themselves!) to do it.

How does cultivating the art of love work? More slowly than you might think—that is to say, step by step; in six steps, to be precise:

Gaining female knowledge about female desire

Knowing one's own experience and taking it seriously

Becoming connected and being in love

Arriving in one's own body

Bringing heart and mind together

Playing and practicing (the main content of this book)

You will find these themes woven throughout *Tantric Sex for Women.*

In addition to practice, the further development of adult sexuality occasionally also requires conscious concentration and sometimes even discipline.

What are these business-world terms doing here in the realm of desire? In our pleasure- and ecstasy-hostile society in general, in the busyness of our everyday lives, in the broad emotional range of our romantic relationships, affairs, and flirtations, there are any number of external, disruptive factors that can destroy a nice atmosphere in no time—especially in the phase of beginning arousal. Even harder to deal with are the internal disruptive factors, in the form of stressful thoughts, evaluations, judgments, plans, etc. *Turning these external and internal disruptions of your love-play into simple incidental occurrences is an absolute skill that can be learned with patience, calmness, concentration, discipline, and an appetite for ecstasy.*

Many women wait for years for the moment at which, with the help of psychotherapy, meditation, interior design according to feng shui, perfect musical accompaniment, and of course a sensitive, perfect lover, they will finally be able to react calmly and cheerfully to disturbances of any kind, to integrate them into the rhythms of their breath, or to cleverly prevent them. Well, that can take time. I, on the other hand, decided one day not to wait until I was on my deathbed (who knows, maybe distractions would win the upper hand there, too?), but rather to try to cultivate my own plea-sure—even if it didn't always work out perfectly. The knowledge I gained in this way, sometimes systematically, sometimes "on the side," is what I would like to share here—spiced up with a wink to the untamable, wild woman and her love of playing.

How to Read This Book

Take a little undisturbed time for yourself; find a comfortable reading po-sition; maybe pour yourself a yummy drink; and above all tap into your childlike curiosity, your adolescent joy in experiments, and your adult de-sires.

This is not a book that needs to be read from front to back—it should inspire you to follow your inner chaos, your curiosity, the flow of your own energy. This is especially true for the games and exercises, which contain both longer and shorter suggestions for how to obtain small ec-stasies in your everyday life. The exercises start in Chapter 3. Before that, Chapter 1 introduces tantra in the context of women's sexuality and Chap-ter 2 reviews the topic of "arriving at home in your own body"—or, to state it more dryly, the anatomy and physiology of the sexual response.

Some of the exercises are designed for the solo lover, and many others are for partners. The exercises are loosely grouped into chapters on, for ex-ample, fantasies, massages, and meditations, to name but a few. The rituals featured in Chapter 8 will give you an idea of the spiritual range that can develop on the playing field of wild-tender pleasure. An Appendix on les-bian sexuality and a section in Chapter 2 on the joys of creative solo sex show how female sexuality can be developed in exclusively female encoun-ters and reflections. An Appendix on sexual energy as a healing force offers a look at the potential restorative pleasures of love-play. Finally, a Re-sources section suggests musical choices that might accompany your prac-ticing and playing with the exercises. It also contains a suggested reading list and resources for playthings and sensual things.

Because this is a book for women, most of the exercises contain in their names and in their activities a specific focus on women's experiences and women's bodies. For example, exercises like "Groaning yoni and laughing belly" (*yoni* is the Sanskrit word for the female genitalia) don't include corresponding language referring to the male anatomy. Likewise, exercises such as "Letting the being in the female lap speak" don't offer alternative activities or interpretations involving men's experiences or male archetypes. And often the pronouns used in the exercises default to the feminine "she" or "her." Does this mean readers are precluded from sharing these love games with a male partner? Absolutely not. Although the book does not give specific suggestions for sexual encounters with men or for mixed-sex tantra sex (there already is enough informative literature available on those topics), with a little imagination and creativity it would be easy enough to substitute male experiences, attitudes, archetypes, and anatomy for the female ones described herein. As the subtitle says, women of all sexual orientations—and their partners—can enjoy and benefit from the book. And men who read it and play with the exercises are likely to gain valuable insight into women and women's sexuality, making them more sensitive and skilled lovers.

Tantric Sex for Women is designed to foster female self-knowledge. My hope is that it encourages women to think (once again) about their sexuality in a playful and pleasurable way, and to differentiate and cultivate it. This is not a book about sexual problems or sex therapy. Neither is it a book about romantic love. Instead, I want to encourage the reader to experiment playfully with herself and others. In addition, I would like to give—particularly to women who are (still) shy about joining a tantra workshop, or who would rather try it out alone—a small insight into the wide variety of ways in which one can further develop one's own sexuality, cultivate it, and even use it to reach meditative states.

And, finally, I would like to mention how wonderful it has been for me as a lesbian to write a book in which women's sexuality is (for a change) in the foreground. I want to encourage every woman to use these suggestions for herself and to make them fit her own particular situation. Let's enjoy what we have in common!

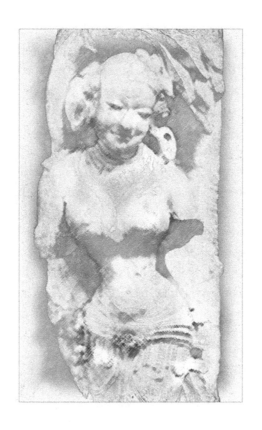

CHAPTER I

The Wisdom of Tantra for Women

GAINING FEMALE KNOWLEDGE ABOUT
FEMALE DESIRE

*T*antra is one way—which I personally find wonderful—to experience love and sexuality as being connected. It is a way to give sexuality, as an expression of love, room for cultivation and refinement. The word *tantra* means network, connection, web, and expansion. It is a word from the language of weavers, and it represents the weft, the string that is pulled through all the warp strings, binding them together.

Tantra means the complete acceptance and weaving together of all our feelings (even the so-called "negative" ones), and the forging of creative bonds with other people. This includes liberation from the prison of polarities and transcendence of social and physical boundaries. It also means beginning with what we have and then expanding it in the direction of our possibilities. In tantric rituals we activate, honor, celebrate, and cultivate our sexual power. We lead it through the inner flute of the individual chakras up to our crown (see Chapter 2) and are thereby able to create a balance between spirit and material, intellect and emotion. That is to say, we dissolve polarities. (The dissolution of polarities by consciously connecting them is a topic very dear to me, since even as a young girl with an "overdose of Catholicism" I had a great longing for a connection between sexuality and spirituality, below and above, inside and outside, between myself and the world.)

Tantra is, for example:

a fine web of tender connection

a dance between the polarities

ecstatic abundance in the everyday

a feast of the senses

finding sense in sensuality

a queen's path to the power of love

a key to the heart

a sweet condensation of passion

the most challenging and fastest way to enlightenment

a medium for the adoration of women

passionate movement and sweet stillness

expanding between heaven and earth to our true size

the cultivation of our love energy beyond old relationship models

a way to heal our sexuality

the constant birth of new life force

the joy of submitting to life

a multiplicity of forms of ecstasy

the possibility to transform existential fears

the power of the quiet encounter

a fleeting experience of eternity

self-love in connection with other self-lovers

a gentle or stormy way to help stretch boundaries

playful swimming in the ocean of desire

a meditation on love

luxurious food for the skin

experiencing the unity of uterus and cosmos

the restoration of female dignity

letting yourself be enchanted by the female scent

the way of the lotus blossom through the mud into the light

Practically speaking, this means that, within a secure, respectful framework and a creative, loving atmosphere, we will begin to activate our sexual power and to reveal the potential of our ecstatic energy through physical exercises, massages, breathing processes, "encounter" games, and touching our pleasure centers. You will find examples of all these activities, and more, in this book. By dealing playfully with this ecstatic energy we learn to hold it, to steer it in various directions, and to let it flow more freely. Particularly good, and developed especially for our Western sensibilities, is Margot Anand's variation on tantra, SkyDancing.

The heart is the most important place for the transformation of physical-emotional energy into spiritual energy. When we connect our sexual energy (in the narrow sense of the word) to the love of the heart, the way is made clear for a third form of energy: mental and spiritual energy. This is the form of energy that flows most gently, most permeably, most quickly through our life-field; it can connect us to others both subtly and intensely, and it is often the foundation for the creation of new ideas or life goals. When sexual energy reaches our spirit by way of the heart, we are able to experience our ecstatic capabilities—for example, in the form of deep feelings of joy, clear visions, feelings of love for ourselves and others, and openings and connections to cosmic energy. From there, in return, we are able to develop a spirituality that is close to life and can be experienced directly. The way of the heart facilitates a joining of sexuality and spirituality that is actually always present. Happiness, therefore, has in reality arrived long ago. We can relax and trust that we will find it again somehow.

When these joyful experiences contrast with the many forms of repression present in a woman-hostile and ecstasy-hostile society, crises must result (for example, when we notice how hard it is in the everyday world to create the conditions necessary for having these feelings). These crises can be conquered through an increased overall energy level, through strong connections from a desiring woman to another person via erotic feelings, and through a deep understanding of ourselves and our world. This happens in a process that I understand as follows: the development of a self-aware, self-contained, and self-sufficient femininity, one that is less and less dependent on outside acknowledgment and is formed more and more by loving encounters and relationships in a broad space and at a tender pace.

Origins of Tantra

Tantric rites began in the Zami cult, a woman-centered sexual cult founded in India by women belonging to a secret sect, as a system of worshiping the yoni. *Yoni* is the Sanskrit name for the female genitalia, with all its little erogenous parts: clitoris, labia, mons veneris, vagina, G-spot, womb, etc. However, *yoni* is much more than an anatomical term, and that's why I prefer it to other names for the same body parts. It is the holy place of female desire, the lap that births new life, and the praiseworthy location of a woman's deepest power. In the allegedly three-thousand-year-old Zami cult, which aimed to reach spiritual, divine planes, sexual exercises were passed on from the older women to the younger ones for the growth of female power. This conclusion is drawn from traditional depictions of women in sexually unambiguous poses and writings, from which we can also conclude—as the Indian archaeologist Giti Thadani has proven—that it must have been a highly pleasurable form of learning.

In the end, the Zami cult was apparently stopped by the rising patriarchy, insofar as the women were forbidden, under pain of extreme torture (such as physical mutilation that included the hacking off of feet), to pass their knowledge along. Later, only a few secret terms indicated these cultic origins; for example, the heart's center was called "the breasts of the sister," and the meditating spirit, which today often has a masculine association, was called "the mother's lap." This means that even in earliest tantric ages, female powers included not only the biological ability to give birth but also the ability to create intellectual life. The two abilities were not seen as separate from one another, but rather were worshiped as the female mystery and were the basis of the belief that the origin of all life is female—including the first images of divinity and the first representations of couples.

With the development of Buddhism, Hinduism, and other foundations of tantrism, new perspectives and valuations of women and men arose, all the way up to the clearly patriarchal representations found in today's Western-influenced tantrism—for example, the tantric melting position of Shiva (or Buddha), the male god, as a big, self-contained figure, and Shakti (or his Dakini, the embodiment of female divinity who sits on him) as a tiny figure of a woman. In the sense of the yin-yang principle, it is said that every woman can integrate the male side—with the image of an inner beloved, embodied by her actual beloved—into her inner identity through a fusion of energy. (For men, correspondingly, the reverse is true.) Still, the starting point is that of a polarity. The old patriarchal principle is at work here, according to which opposites are created so that they can be integrated. A consensus is reached about the alleged archetypal opposition between men and women, and these placatingly simple polar qualities are constantly reideologized and respiritualized. So a quality like aggressiveness is more likely to be connoted as masculine than connected, say, with the female archetype of the Amazon. This polarized thinking, then, reduces us to the usual societal women's roles from which we can then be "rescued" by fusion—either directly with men or with masculine forms of energy.

Many feminists who are usually open to impulses that further their own sexual development are concerned by the recent trend toward tantric workshops and groups, since even in the outer structure of rituals, heterosexist prejudices and restrictions are visible. If, however, I do not stay on the surface, but rather delve into tantric atmospheres, exercises, and worlds of experience that are shaped by female perception, feeling, and thinking, I can, as a woman, experience a strengthening, a connection with other women, an integration with little-lived parts of myself, and a transformation of material energy into spiritual. This works to strengthen women, to connect women, and to interweave women, and it promotes the anarchic strength of our sexual energy. Of course, embracing these notions requires accepting only that which promotes our own growth and the growth of female strength and freedom—a conscious tightrope walk between accepting and distancing, between context-bound enjoyment and recognizing premature definitions about "feminine nature" (making gender assumptions), etc. Still, even an initially very cautious tightrope walk can turn into a satisfying walk in the clouds or a wonderful journey of discovery to a distant land that doesn't correspond to the classic measurements of normative sexuality.

What Possibilities for Growth Can Today's Tantra Offer Us Women?

Tantra can offer women a way to energize themselves and to take on a self-aware vitality—not just out of aggression and to overcome fear, but from mutually experienced desire and sensuality. This way of being together has, in my mind, fallen too much into the background amidst the necessities of battle in the newer women's movements.

It's high time we showed solidarity, not just in the fight against something or in suffering from something, but *in the creation of maximal pleasure and in the expansion of this pleasure in all directions!* It goes without saying that our efforts along these lines will not proceed without fear, mistrust, the working through of violent experiences, and the devaluation of desire and sensuality.

Tantra offers a way out of this. All the hurts, all the suffering, all the feelings of powerlessness and guilt can be experienced and expressed. The goal of tantric energy processes is not, however, to indulge in these feelings, but instead to dedicate ourselves consciously to the other side: that of desire, sensuality, and spiritual growth. The point is to restore a sacred space and healing power to our sexuality—capacities it has, in fact, always had. The fact that this path sometimes contains stumbling blocks should not prevent us from setting out on it.

Whenever I look at old tantric writings from India or Tibet, they make the feminine central to the culture—giving the woman an important position, even elevating her to a cosmic force, a personal embodiment of extrapersonal divinity. There are various goddesses (such as Tara, Kali, and Baubo) who embody different aspects of femininity; calling on them can activate these aspects or energy forms within women.

The basic idea passed on to us by these traditions is that divinity is not outside of us but is *within* each person, *within* each woman. It can be experienced in our moments of greatest ecstasy, which are reached especially through sexual unity with others in a circle of simultaneous desire. This lets us experience the source of our own pleasure as coming from within us rather than from a partner. So sexuality becomes the sanctified earthly path to our own divine nature, since it can bind together the planes of physicality, emotionality, communication, intellectuality, and spirituality as an all-encompassing and foundational life force.

Finding the courage to form our own lives according to our knowledge and nature is a life's work for each of us, since psychic growth comes much more slowly than our intellectual insights into women's power and women's autonomy. So let's take our time and use it well! *Use* in this context means

that I will see this time as a time for living, a space that I will fill with encounters, feelings, and my vitality, until finally I spend my living time in a
way that is my own, thus finding meaning in my life. On this point tantra
differs from psychotherapy. Tantric fantasy-"work" or other self-discovery
"work" does allow old problems, hurts, disturbances, and conflicts to be
"felt out" and partially even expressed, but the focus is on the search for an
individual desire for life and its foundations. Resistance—for example, in
the form of drifting off into old reactions of pain and sorrow—is reduced by either a playful approach or creating structural boundaries. Desire is emphasized mainly by supporting the energy level of the individual,
but also by creating a sensual-aesthetic ambiance and introducing tempting
experiments, and through bodily interventions such as stretching, relaxation, and letting oneself be more permeable. What is important is to *allow*
all the feelings that are tangible at that moment but not to get *caught up* in
specific feelings. Instead, observe them and let go of them again, and transform individual feelings into the next highest plane through chaneling your
energies higher. On the social level, this means neither running around au-
tonomously without connections to other people nor projecting your own
interests onto others (e.g., men). Instead, it means simply being able to exist in the knowledge of the power of your own female eroticism, being
self-sufficient, self-contained, and open to encounters that serve your own
growth.

Tara: A Sexual Role Model for Women

Women need sexual role models because sexual energy can be so strong
that it is frightening. Role models help change this combination of fear
and desire into curiosity and play. For many of us, images of sexual
women as we know them—that is, from childhood—are ambivalent or
negative, since sex was coupled with devaluation, disrespect, possession, or
violence. We may also have had role models—whether older sisters, the
Virgin Mary, or movie stars—who were so desexualized that the desire to
emulate them ("good") and the wish to experiment with sexual feelings
("bad") were fundamentally opposed.

I am familiar with this stubborn resistance to everyone and everything
presented as a sexual role model; I wasn't able to see myself in them, and I

found the subtle or even obvious pressure to conform despicable. But it's not easy to create a solid female sexual identity solely out of one's own current relationships, a few honest responses, and one's own games of trial and error. It seems more useful to look for images and role models who are more than personal, who embody neither the cultural pressure to conform nor are as distant as today's beauty icons, who are general enough to be a good projection surface for our own wishes and longings, and who can embody a woman in all her dimensions (physical, emotional, intellectual, spiritual). For example, goddess figures. But be careful: Many goddesses are bound up with patriarchal contexts and, accordingly, have limited female-sexual identities or are dependent on male gods. Still, I believe in the saying by the philosopher Erich Neumann, adapted for us women: "If you take away the women's goddess, you take away their identity!"

I find this maxim particularly apt because women's power, even in matriarchal societies—societies shaped by female genealogy and power—was weakened by the fact that the growing patriarchy gave goddess figures a lesser or negative meaning, or they even disappeared altogether, to be replaced by male gods.

In order to prevent our contemporary sexuality from being further "demonized," devalued, ignored, controlled, or alienated by the male gaze, we need pictures, role models, and projections in which our sexuality can be seen clearly—as it is seen by the female gaze. With the "overdose of Catholicism" I received as a child, newer versions of the Virgin Mary (which ask, for example, whether she might be acknowledged as a goddess in her own right, rather than merely playing her role as an asexual Madonna and mother of God) were out of the question. So I looked into many other religions and cultures, and finally I found Tara, the "Mother of Tibet," the great liberator of women, the free woman who promised to be incarnated as a woman again and again for the good of all women, for the good of all beings. Tara's most important feature for me, though, is that she is not venerated as being outside of us, but rather is seen as the embodiment of all women, so that calling on her various major qualities (generosity, sympathy, patience, submission, quick action when necessary) means activating these energies in myself, rather than looking for them somewhere else. Furthermore, what I like about this figure—especially the

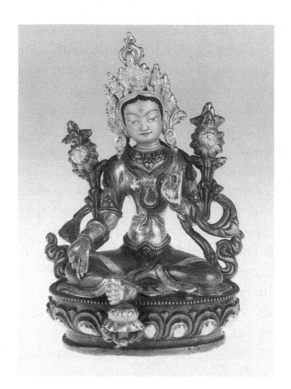

**Figure 1.
The Goddess
Tara.**

"Green Tara," who is seen as the "goddess of great sympathy and fearless action"—is that she is sitting on her lotus blossom, sensual and relaxed, with only one foot; the other is stretched out as if ready to "spring into the world," where with her great sympathy she can act to liberate and empower all beings. This readiness to quickly change the state of affairs is, for me, the ideal of a sexually *and* politically active woman.

Below, as an example of an image of female identity, are the wonderful major characteristics of Tara within us. They can liberate us from oppression (more details on this topic can be found in the books of Sylvia Wetzel and Pema-Dorje), and here I have reformulated them for the purpose of liberating female sexuality:

I. *Generosity* is the ability to think not only about yourself, but also to look beyond yourself. Being generous means having a big heart—one that can bear much, be deeply touched, give everyone room, and encounter itself and others with warmth, sympathy, and goodwill. This creates an all-encompassing certainty that can make you relaxed and calm, and can help you keep sight of the "bigger picture" during the turbulence of life. Generosity is the ability to give yourself and others love from the fullness of your heart.

2. *Patience* means being relaxed—being able to wait, staying calm, and giving yourself the necessary playing room for development. Patience creates space—living space, breathing space, space to develop. It is the opposite of fearful defensive maneuvers and the rigid "no!" in response to everything that is new or different. Patience means showing forbearance for ourselves, for the beloved who is so darned "different," and for all other beings.

3. *Integrity* means not harming anyone and not hurting anyone; respecting another's desires; not taking anything that is not given; and not tolerating any untruths, but rather conquering illusions and fighting for truth. In other words, it means the creation of inner conditions for an active, pleasurable, free female life.

4. *Strength of will* and *diligence* mean awakening your own energy and acting creatively to open yourself up to cosmic energy. This includes the conscious decision to practice (e.g., to repeat a meditation so many times that it becomes a given in your everyday routine) and to overcome internal defensive hurdles (e.g., the fear of new things).

5. *Kindness* and *gentleness* mean being kind to yourself in order to experience Tara within yourself. This is the great turning point in your life. It does not mean being taken advantage of, inhibiting your aggressions, and being a passive victim. What is important is becoming gentler (particularly toward yourself); feeling your own hunger for light, warmth, and goodness; and rediscovering your inner gentleness in the darkness of your own heart and letting yourself be touched by it. This creates another, self-evident network among your varying emotional states and between you and the people around you. By being kind to myself (and my so-called weaknesses) and to others, and by having an open and gentle aura, I can develop a web of giving and taking, one that is marked by inner wealth, sovereignty, and freedom.

6. *Wisdom* is related to being aware and to experiencing reason in this way. It is a gradual, drawn-out process of becoming and growing. The conscious spirit is the decisive organ here; meditation or sexuality in its spiritual dimension are the ways and means. Wisdom overcomes all "opposite" poles and recognizes the "unity of multiplicity." From this place comes a liberation from deceptions and illusion, from battles and tensions and rigidity. Wisdom illuminates the here and now and helps us transcend the situation at hand. The way to wisdom is through stillness.

These qualities, which have been present in us all along, are most easily summoned by remembering situations in which we have already experienced them. In order to strengthen them and make them a more conscious part of our person, we sing the Tara mantra:

OM TARE TUTTARE TURE SOHA

Its meaning can be translated approximately as follows: "With that holy sound that constantly rings out around the world, the sound of those meditating in all languages, we call you, O Tara, whose wonderful qualities are awakened in us, driving away fears and causing joy, for the good of all beings, let it be so."

However, silence, as a space in which the kind wisdom of Tara develops within me, does not necessarily exist just because I want it to. Sometimes we need violent movement, a loud racket, emotional uproar, or a lot of interpersonal contacts and activities before we grow tired of them and can try to enter inner and outer spaces of stillness. Furthermore, Western-oriented tantra often begins loudly, expansively, and gregariously, until the consciously perceived energy grows more refined, still, and intimate in the exercises and rituals.

The goal of tantra, then, is a meditation on love that does not pass over sexual desire, but goes along with it and through it. From there, advanced tantrikas (all women who practice tantra in some form or another) can, for example, experience orgasmic highs without any physical contact, or from very little contact can enter into ecstatic states that unleash enormous creative potential. This is the inner Tara, she who liberates us from old inhibitions and boundaries that have become unnecessary—a free woman who draws her wisdom from her desire and uses it to do her work in the world.

Principles of Cultivated, Self-Willed Sexuality

So that the reader can follow my way of thinking, let me briefly restate from the Introduction my basic understanding of women's sexuality: *Female sexuality is the totality of that which women imagine to be sexuality, even if they only feel and experience a fragment thereof.* Now let's take it a step further. To get the most out of the exercises outlined in this book, it is a good idea to embrace—or at least to become open to embracing—certain basic tenets of what I would call a "self-willed sexuality." By opening yourself to the following principles, you take the first steps toward claiming your sexuality and all its life-changing power as your own. In addition, let yourself engage in much discussion about these principles with others, especially about the concrete steps involved in putting them into practice for yourself.

* You are the source of your sexuality—not your partner or your environment. It is completely up to you whether you enjoy yourself or not, or whether you have a good sexual experience or not.

* Trust that your beloved can take care of herself or himself.

* Concentrate on your inner perception and observe subtle changes in your breathing; breathing broadens your feelings. Breathing deeply while making love helps you accept momentary sensations. Sexual breathing turns your whole body into a pleasure organ.

* Allow yourself to give in to the moment. Feelings and sensations are conditions that "happen" from one moment to the next. Allow yourself to express every soft and loud sound, every small and large movement. Allow yourself to flow and to melt into yourself, into your partner, into the world.

* Try to accept and appreciate yourself just as you are. Allow yourself to feel good, and grant yourself permission to have "crazy" or "superior" feelings.

✳ Develop a friendly relationship with yourself—become your own best friend. Do just as much for yourself as you do for your beloved. If this is not (yet) possible for you, you can occasionally "pretend" that you are deeply in love with yourself and that your self-love is already wonderfully cultivated.

✳ You can change the context in which you place your experience so that it becomes fun, pleasurable, and joyful. Be prepared to experience *all* sensations as pleasurable—even so-called "negative" feelings.

✳ Allow yourself to try out new things: shaking yourself, breathing more intensely, laughing a lot, tickling the other person, becoming mystical. Crying, screaming, and laughing are natural ways to express the intensity of your sexual energy. Do whatever you want. In sexuality, there is no "right" or "wrong." There is only a common striving for desire. Whatever pleases you *and* your partner is allowed.

✳ If you experiment with your sexuality in different situations and contexts, you will make different discoveries; try it outdoors, dressed, dressed up, naked, in forbidden places....

✳ Let yourself be orgasmic. To be orgasmic is to be able to give in, to swing, to flow, to dissolve into something larger than yourself—an ability developed while you relaxed, floated, and merged in your mother's womb. If you want to feel this old cosmic, oceanic sensation again, you just need to concentrate on it, breathe deeply, and relax.

✳ Allow yourself to be orgasmic and ecstatic in more ways than one. Being orgasmic does not necessarily have to do with sex; it means finding intense pleasure in whatever is happening and feeling that pleasure. You can be orgasmic without having an orgasm. You can turn orgasmic feelings into ecstasies by letting the fire of your lust smolder and by not hindering its spreading.

✳ Ecstasy is a natural—and actually lasting—state of maximal pleasure. And (sexual) pleasure is the most expansive feeling we have.

There is always more pleasure, more delight, more ecstasy than you feel right at this moment. Finding "heaven on earth" is simply a matter of concentration, broadening, and development.

✳ If you are highly sexually charged and can't come as quickly as usual, relax into this excitement without doing anything. Conscious, alert inaction is the basis and ideal state of tantric (and most other) meditations. Inaction is the love nest of Lady Happiness and her partner, Lady of Tender Times.

✳ The more often you play with your sexual energy and the more you practice calling, steering, packaging, and expanding it, the easier it will be for you to experience positive feelings and desires, and the more your body will integrate them and respond with increasingly positive reactions.

✳ Do whatever is necessary to bring yourself to the point where everything feels good.

These principles might seem simple and self-evident at first sight. However, I know from my own experience how delicate and easily disrupted their implementation is. Therefore, the exercises offered in this book are designed to pave the way to pleasure and even more pleasure, to get the stumbling blocks out of the way (or to help us let them passively-lasciviously pass us by), and, of course, to offer a sense of the wide space of orgasmic ecstasies.

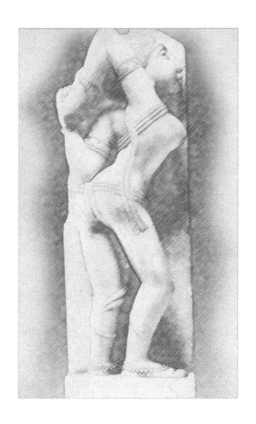

≈ CHAPTER 2 ≈

Setting the Stage

ARRIVING AT HOME IN YOUR OWN BODY

*T*he ways to pleasure, arousal, and ecstasy are as diverse as women themselves are. So let us leave behind the old norms, the supposedly statistically proven orgasm curves, and other reductions of the multiple ways in which women can achieve sexual happiness, and draw our attention to our own reality!

In this chapter I first address women's most important pleasure organs. I also seize the opportunity to do away with old misapprehensions about female anatomy and physiology. Then I talk about different forms of orgiastic energy and ecstasy. A short summary of chakra teachings follows (an understanding of which makes it easier to do the exercises for transforming sexual energy into spiritual energy), and finally there is a section about sexual self-love, which I like to call the queen of all forms of love (even though no form can actually be replaced by another).

I hope the reader will find confirmation here of her own experience, and that she will also find, in place of dry theory, a few moist suggestions for playfully exploring the physical as well as the spiritual sides of pleasure.

What Does Desire Do, and Where?

In principle, every body part can be an erogenous zone—and can set off orgasms, too. With the appropriate stance and attitude, every woman can create orgasms *through purely spiritual means* (for example, with sexual fantasies or simply by concentrating on her ecstatic capabilities); therefore, a woman's sexual satisfaction can be independent from others, and even from her own "handiwork." But the easiest way to reach sexual arousal is through direct stimulation of the different erogenous zones, which, once awakened, generally tend to combine their individual sensations with those from other zones to create a greater wave of sexual energy. I briefly introduce each of them here.

THE NIPPLES

These peaks of the breasts, which stand up during arousal, are clearly organs of sexual arousal (unlike lips, earlobes, big toes, or inner thighs, which

I would classify as erogenous zones). This is undoubtedly the case when their stimulation can be felt in an energetic connection with the clitoris and vagina—a connection that can express itself as a reflective pulsing (as though a delicate pleasure-information superhighway lay between the nipples and the clitoris, labia, and vagina, through which even the smallest movements run back and forth) or as a swelling, damp and receptive. The nipples are also the "receptive antennae" of the female body, lying closest to the heart, so that stroking them opens the heart a little, giving feelings of love and attraction a palpable location. This phenomenon is of particular importance in spiritual orgasms, since the heart chakra, the energy funnel of the entire chest region, represents the "switchboard" where sexual energy becomes spiritual, where physical forms of love become intellectual. This means that in the clear consciousness of the heart level there lies the "secret" of transforming material energy and reaching a further, "higher" level of consciousness.

THE YONI

By this tantric word, I mean all the sexually excitable parts of the "lower lust level" of the female body: the outer pleasure forest (or, in old age, the clearing) with its external G-spot at the base of the Venus mountain, the clitoris, the inner and outer labia, the vagina with its erectile tissue and its various pleasure points, the uterus and its opening, the perineum, and even the anus (see Figure 2 on page 27).

Why am I adopting a Sanskrit word, *yoni,* from a totally different culture and tradition? Words like *cunt* or *pussy* have a negative emotional connotation for many women, and a word like *vulva* is often used only to mean what is visible from the outside. Some of the nice-sounding, flowery words are imprecise, and medical jargon is completely out of the question. What is beautiful about the word *yoni* is not just its sound, but also the deeper meaning of its symbolism. It describes not only the entire female genital system, but also the universal lap: female energy in and of itself (seen as divine), which is honored in a sexual encounter. This fits in with my theory that there is really only one kind of energy, in the form of oscillations and smaller parts, that gets its color from the organ where it is created or toward which it is directed. Yoni energy becomes colored as sexual energy, for example; it takes on the qualities of this organ until it is directed elsewhere or is spread out or transformed. I see the principles of this energy theory reflected in the word *yoni*.

But rather than complaining about the shortcomings of our language (after all, we now have Laura Méritt's *Sexcapades* and Eve Ensler's *Vagina Monologues*), let me inspire you with a few names for a woman's pleasure center, dreamed up by the participants in one of my first tantric playshops:

bearded Venus	*pomegranate*	*little chamber*
witches' honey	*honey mouth*	*sweetie*
butterfly	*playmate*	*wild creek*
South Sea pearl	*greedy dragoness*	*wildcat*
pearl box	*magic mussel*	*magic fold*
dream gate	*source of joy*	*oyster*
paradise gate	*fig*	*pleasure gorge*
lust cave	*goddess flesh*	*little pleasure well*
pleasure forest	*love nectar*	*nest of madness*
poppy flower	*witches' broom bristles*	*little Niagara Falls*
lust grotto	*dewdrop*	*wishing gate*
Venus garden	*sweet snail*	*fairy harp*
passion flower	*forest glade*	*Tara temple*

Now for the individual parts of the yoni:

The clitoris

This is made up not just of that little pearl, with or without its hood, and the top edge of the inner labia; it continues with a short shaft and a long shank within the body that stretches into the vagina in a Y shape and surrounds the urinary tract. (The arbitrarily defined length of the shaft determines whether a woman is labeled female or androgynous.) Sensitivity to direct or indirect, strong or gentle touch varies widely and generally changes over the course of arousal; for many women, for example, sensitivity grows

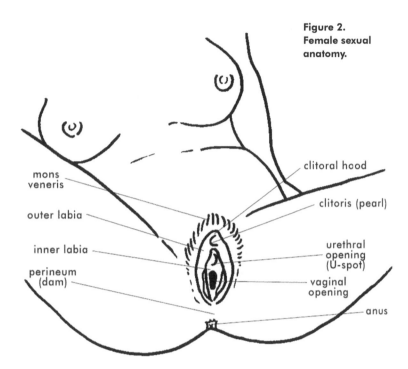

**Figure 2.
Female sexual
anatomy.**

mons
veneris

outer labia

inner labia

perineum
(dam)

clitoral hood

clitoris (pearl)

urethral
opening
(U-spot)

vaginal
opening

anus

with each orgasm until the clitoris is hypersensitive. As a woman gets older (especially after menopause, when lubrication can decrease), her skin—especially the pearl of the clitoris and most other mucous membranes—becomes more sensitive, so that it usually feels more pleasurable and less "rough" to stimulate the clitoris with the help of a water-soluble lubricant, just as a full-body massage using body oil is usually more pleasant than one without. Orgasms resulting from direct or nearly direct stimulation of the clitoris are more explosively directed outward and for many women can be repeated frequently over a short period of time.

Directly below the clitoris, at its root (the frenulum), is where most (but not all) women's inner labia meet. Many nerve endings come together in this little fold of skin, which means that direct or indirect contact can be very pleasurable.

The labia

As varied as the orchid family, these form the kissing mouth of the yoni.

They protect our innermost pleasure organs and open readily when kissed and touched gently. The more aroused we are, the better their circulation is and the larger they grow. In contrast to the hairy, fleshy outer labia, the inner lips—no matter what their shape—are usually slightly damp; they usually like to be stroked, kneaded, and nibbled, and they like to slurp up fingers and other things. Having them caressed is not always highly arousing, but doing so usually improves sensitivity everywhere in yoni-land.

The U-spot

This least-known pleasure point is part of the urinary tract's erectile tissue (the urethra, which is why it's called the U-spot). It is generally found next to the urinary opening—in many women, two to three centimeters below the clitoris. Because of this, it is often stimulated "by accident" along with the clitoris, but when it is directly stimulated, it has its own sweet quality of energy, one that contributes more toward implosive, although outwardly stiller, orgasms. The more it's pampered, the more it becomes raised and can be seen as a fingertip-sized nub. It may change position slightly (for example, through muscle contractions just before an orgasm) but will remain near the urinary tract and—together with the G-spot—can induce a stream of joy: female ejaculation.

The G-spot

Although many women have found it for themselves, the G-spot is named after its official "discoverer," a certain Mr. Gräfenberg. This pleasure point, which is sometimes a palpable nub and sometimes a whole surface of little nubs, is found under the urinary tract opening, somewhere along the front wall of the vagina (the exact location varies from woman to woman). It, too, becomes more alert and sensitive the more it is stimulated. A woman who is looking for it for the first time can usually recognize it by her strong need to pee when the spot is touched, even if her bladder is empty. That's the right spot. And if she doesn't run right to the bathroom but instead relaxes into the feeling, she will experience the spread of a pleasurable sweetness throughout her entire pelvis. One woman called her G-spot her "singing point" because when it was stimulated, she felt like a tender, sweet song was spreading through her pelvis and making her happy in a softly swinging way. For some women, the excited glands in the erectile tissue of the G-spot create an ejaculate—from a few drops to about two quarts of a watery, odorless liquid that is not to be confused with urine—that can flow out onto a layer of towels atop a plastic sheet in her love nest, carefully laid out ahead of time, or over her sexual partner.

The M-spot

This spot (which I've named *M* as in "mmmmm," something especially yummy) can only be felt after at least one of the other kinds of orgasms—orgasmic pleasuring of the pearl, G-spot, or U-spot, or, more rarely, after an earlier nipple orgasm. The spot lies just below the mouth of the uterus and, felt from the front, is a little behind the bottom end of the uterus. It can be felt when the vagina lifts up, forming a kind of tent with the uterus that is sometimes called the vaginal roof. At the inner peak of that little tent lies this pleasure point, with an energy quality that is best described as a tender flow of hot firewater. This firewater has the tendency to spread upward to the heart or the third eye and feels like liquid joy. It is most easily pleasured by a long-fingered partner who can tap, ring, or vibrate it softly and constantly. It's harder to reach with your own fingers or a dildo (even a so-called G-spot dildo), but a good, strong vibrator can stimulate it indirectly. Instead of a short climax, it creates the feeling of a long, dizzying high point—the kind you'd experience just before you lift off and fly.

The perineum (dam)

The perineum is usually the lowest point of the entire yoni region when a woman is in a squatting position. It is located between the vaginal opening and anus. If I want to glide into my beloved's pleasure tunnel, I find it only polite to knock here first and see if I'm allowed in. When it is stimulated/awakened or pulled upward as you inhale, it strengthens and activates the vaginal opening and can make entering the lust tunnel exciting and arousing. As the lowermost part of the root chakra, its stimulation can create a sensation of general vitality and earthy power.

The anus

This body part—often disparaged because of its excremental function and because many of us are raised to be highly concerned about cleanliness, but that also has a thin wall to the internal G-spot—is not simply the entrance for a visit to the two rosettes (sphincter muscles) with their own pleasure qualities (which vary according to the woman and her mood). Just before its entrance, at the lowest part of the coccyx (tailbone), lies the kundalini point—the pleasure point that, when tapped or vibrated, can create a delicate, snakelike feeling of pleasure from the lowermost point of the spinal column all the way up to the head, energizing the whole body and gladdening the soul. When stimulating the sensitive anus region, practicing safer-sex techniques is especially important. This includes, for example, making sure a finger that has been inside the anus does not touch the vagina until the finger has been thoroughly washed, to prevent bacteria from being transmitted. In order to prevent unwanted pain from infringing on pleasure, the generous use of lubricants is recommended—the water-soluble kind is best, because it can be washed off easily afterward. For the inner anal canal and the nearby intestinal region, oil-based creams like Vaseline are useful. (Caution: Petroleum-based products can make latex gloves or condoms and silicone toys porous, and thus should not enter the vagina.) Above all, use only extremely short fingernails in order to protect the injury-prone rectal walls (especially if you like to have several fingers or a whole hand inside you).

The PC muscle

The *pubococcygeus* or *pubococcygeal muscle group,* which is often called the *PC muscle* for short, is a part of the pelvic musculature. It stretches between the pubic bone and the coccyx, surrounds the vaginal opening, and crosses over the perineum in two bands like a figure eight (see Figure 3 on page 31). This pleasure muscle can be consciously flexed, relaxed, and pressed. Exercising it improves the circulation of the entire yoni and supports the ability to transpose sexual arousal in an orgiastic way. The better it is trained, the stronger its orgasm-promoting effects will be. In addition, targeted flexing and relaxing can hurl sexual fire upward like glowing lava in a volcanic eruption. (Okay, sometimes it's more like a warm

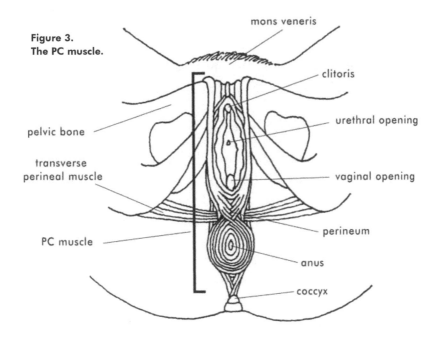

**Figure 3.
The PC muscle.**

mons veneris

clitoris

pelvic bone

urethral opening

transverse
perineal muscle

vaginal opening

PC muscle

perineum

anus

coccyx

flow than molten, flaming lava.) This powerful hurling upward or the more gentle nudging comes from pumping the PC. Here's how: At the beginning of an inward breath (and eventually independent of your breathing), the muscle is energetically tensed and then released, and during the exhale it is pressed downward. This moves (sexual) energy up and down through the intersection between your perineum and the crown of your head. (This is only one of the many PC-muscle exercises that are part of the pelvic training that is described in detail by, for example, Benita Cantieni in her book *Tiger Feeling.*)

THE HEAD

The head is not just a place for the thinking apparatus, for intuition, and for combining perception and feeling. In addition to the sensitive skin areas it houses, in addition to the speaking, singing, and kissing mouth and the hairline, it contains the eyes, ears (which regulate one's sense of balance), and nose, which are important sensory organs for eroticism and sexuality. They lend your inner-body experience a special flavor and make lively contact with your sexual partner possible. So we should at least see the head as one of our erogenous zones rather than obsessing over its intellectual function, which is often distracting and limiting. This does not mean "switching it off" for the benefit of ecstatic sexuality, but instead concentrating on the functions that increase desire.

Orgasm and Ecstasy

An orgasm really has nothing to do with "need," but many women feel enormous pressure to "come," if possible multiple times, in order to prove something to themselves and maybe to their partners. The expectation seems to be to prove that they are (pick one or more) real/mature/ uncomplicated/potent women. On a purely rational level, we distance ourselves from patriarchal standards about orgasm, just as we no longer make the official measurements and definitions of male sexologists our guidelines. But many of us have not yet chased these norms—such as Freud's "mature, vaginal orgasm"—from our souls. Therefore, we are still easily hurt by underestimations and questioning.

Some women have proposed that we come up with our own terminology. A coinage like "orgas-can," say (as opposed to "orgas-must"), sounds less like pressure than permission, but it doesn't really sound like fun and pleasure either. Another possibility is "orgas-yum," but that's a word I find difficult to associate with tenderness, breadth, scope, and melting into love. Still, this kind of term coining has more to do with the desire for the possibility of ecstatic conditions than with fixation on a goal (the famously measurable spasms of the vagina) that others have set for us. As an XXL woman, I am always reminded of the fashion industry's attempt to tailor "one size fits all" clothing to fit every female figure—with the end result being that it doesn't really fit anyone. Many women continue to think that there is only *one* goal in sex, only *one* kind of ecstasy, which is the "right" one because of its size, intensity, depth, duration, whatever. And yet, if we pay close attention and take ourselves seriously, we all basically know that *what's right is what feels really good for us (me)*.

We often reduce the scope of all possible ecstasies to those few seconds that call themselves "orgasm." And some women even deny themselves that kind of ecstasy, reducible to a physical, physiologically measurable event, for a variety of reasons (for example, because their muscular tension is too high or low, or because they define their menstrual period as a sex-free phase). Furthermore, many women don't really know what orgiastic kinds of ecstasy are and how they can be reached. Here, instead of giving exact physiological information that can be looked up elsewhere in many books, I think it's important to mention that only part of this ecstasy has to do with the sharp peak that can be reached through certain techniques that precisely stimulate the clitoris, G-spot, etc. More of it has to do with states of happiness, excitement, emotion, stretching, movement, emptiness, peace, and flowing love. These vary widely according to the individual, depending on her (preexisting) mood, the love that is present in the encounter, the individual's physical condition, and the ability to gain momentum with herself and the other(s).

Gina Ogden has conducted some enlightening research. She asked a large number of women to describe their orgasms and by doing so discovered some of the very complex structures of the orgasmic experience. In the book *Women Who Love Sex,* she describes pleasure, orgasm, and ecstasy as three overlapping energy spheres that can be understood both as a continuum *and* as different shades of one and the same sexual energy. Each of these spheres includes all the levels of the body, soul, spirit, and spirituality. In times of greatest joy, all levels are experienced as one—a fusion with a partner or with oneself and the whole world. In my experience, the most important part of this phenomenon is the momentary dissolving of one's own borders and those of space and time, connected to a burst of energy, an expanding lust for life and love. The moment is usually preceded by total concentration on what feels good and on your love for yourself and/or your partner. The subsequent giving in to the moment and to the sensation of love energy is consciously allowed rather than instinctively kept out. This state can pretty much create itself *as long as we don't hinder the flow of energy, but instead open ourselves wider and more deeply, giving in to all (!) feelings that come up without fixating on keeping them forever or on avoiding them in the future.* This way, an orgasm is more likely to "happen" to us rather than being "created."

✳ SIGNS OF ORGASM LEVELS IN LOVERS

Level	Energized body part	Noticeable reactions
1	lungs	she sighs, breathes heavily, and saliva collects in her mouth
2	heart	loving, longing glances; frequent desire for a French kiss; licking of highly erogenous skin areas; tender sounds
3	spleen, pancreas, and stomach	her muscles are activated; her pelvis makes spontaneous swinging or tipping motions; frequent desire for embraces and stroking
4	kidneys and bladder	her yoni begins to pulsate; love juices flow
5	bones	her limbs and joints grow soft/elastic, especially the hip joint and sometimes, reflexively, the jaw (which is energetically connected to the pelvic floor/perineum; possible desire to bite
6	liver and nerves	she rears up, twists like a snake, and often wants to throw her arms and legs around her partner
7	blood	her blood circulates faster and more visibly; she wants to actively touch her lover or tense up completely; or she experiences aggressive impulses
8	muscles	the tension in her outer muscles relaxes, while the inner ones tighten, and this sometimes also happens in connection with strong movements of the outer muscles and loud noises (screaming, stretched-out moaning, murmuring, jubilation)
9	the whole body	she relaxes completely and experiences a "small death" (i.e., her body can become very still for a moment before smaller or larger wave motions visibly flow through her); she gives in completely and opens herself fully
10	third eye/head	her facial expressions as well as the rest of her body "melt away," that is, a joyful mood spreads through her, over her whole body, and can palpably fill the beloved and the entire room
11	crown	her body lies still, and she feels a "light heaviness" that is sometimes interrupted by single spasms of the whole body or changes in breathing frequency; her experiences of colors, pictures, films, feelings of happiness, emptiness, or transcendence at this point are not as visible—she will have to tell you about them later

The chart on page 34 describes some of the bodily reactions involved in these pleasure processes. The "levels" assigned to these descriptions are simply a convenient, if somewhat arbitrary, numerical way to identify the different areas of the body involved.

The Variety and Diversity of Women's Orgasms

We know of course that women differ from each other in their feelings and physical pleasure organs as much as wild roses differ from one another. Acknowledging unity in diversity is usually easier for us when we have positive terms for what is different and what is shared, and when we attempt to categorize them intellectually—always with the awareness of the old sage who smiles at such efforts and then does what she wants anyway.

For example, the Cherokee Indians have undertaken investigations to differentiate between the types of orgasm experienced by women. (Of course orgasm here is not understood as it is by the "classic" treatises of sexual education, which present it simply in terms of the Gaussian normal curve, but rather as the many forms that women's sexual ecstasy can take.)

In the system described by the Cherokees, the features of the different orgasm types are associated with the characteristics of the four points of the compass. All are connected to the center, and all have spiraling qualities that create themselves anew with every experience. In this approach, the way female sexuality grows is described as a process of differentiation that takes place in encounters and relationships between individuals.

To represent this diversity, ten different categories were formed in which anatomical features correlate with physiological, psychological, and communicative reactions:

1. distance between the pearl (clitoris) and lust grotto (vagina)

2. nature of the little hat of the pearl (hood of the clitoris)

3. nature of the inner labia and relation to outer Venus lips (labia)

4. depth of lust tunnel (vagina)

5. position of the G-spot (Gräfenberg spot), the most sensitive erectile tissue

6. moisture inside the lust cave

7. temperature inside the lust grotto

8. taste of the fluid

9. form of preferred stimulation if orgiastic ecstasy is desired

10. preferred love position for best stimulation

These categories should be understood as subjective research criteria that the Cherokees used when they investigated themselves and others. Based on these criteria, they devised five orgasm "types." To promote better understanding, I changed the descriptions a bit and named them after flowers. My descriptions are presented below. Please note that there can be blends of different orgasm types. This is especially true of women who have the characteristics of "noon flower," which is estimated to be 50–60 percent of women. Each of the other positions accounts for about 5–10 percent of women. (In our European and North American latitudes there are usually more "lilies" and not more than 6 percent are "corn poppies.")

The characteristics can also vary within one type, depending, for example, on a woman's menstrual cycle, sexual activity, diet, and factors relating to mood or stress. Obviously, there are still clear tendencies within the particular orgasm types. Furthermore, low frequencies and depths of orgasm can be changed through the use of exercises described in this book, like Exercise 17, "Gladdening the heart." In other words, these types are not rigidly predefined, but rather are an identification of variety and possibility. Take the following descriptions more as suggestions for reflection, self-investigation, and playing, rather than for evaluating and determining.

THE FIVE ORGASM TYPES

Lily

Point on the compass: north

Element: air

Anatomical characteristics: long, smooth tunnel; clit at the end, with a dis-

tance between clit and vaginal opening of two to three fingers wide; labia and hood formed from the same tissue; inner labia thin; deep cave; G-spot deep inside
Lubrication (wetness): very wet
Temperature in cave: warm
Taste: sweet
Preferences: indirect stimulation of the clit by rubbing the hood; long, slow tuning in; oral sex; hard sucking of the labia; pressing or gliding along the hood; rubbing of mons veneris
Preferred positions: prefers to be on top; crouching (plucking the pearl from behind, or walking into the lust tunnel)

Orchid

Point on the compass: east
Element: water
Anatomical characteristics: many folds in both labia; inner labia overhanging and thick; hoodlike teepee tent; shallow cave; G-spot halfway between uterus and cave entry
Lubrication (wetness): moist but not wet
Temperature in cave: cool
Taste: salty
Preferences: needs a lot of preparation and tuning in; frequent and long rubbing of clit; oral sex; steady rhythm; playing with folds of Venus lips
Preferred positions: spoon position or side by side; seesaw movements and sitting intertwined

Rose

Point on the compass: south
Element: fire
Anatomical characteristics: big, thin, overhanging inner labia, like bat wings; distance between clitoris and vaginal entry several fingers wide; small hood over clit; moderate length of cave; G-spot in the back; uterus often bent
Lubrication (wetness): wet
Temperature in cave: warm to hot
Taste: sweet-salty

Preferences: likes to be noisy when making love; likes sex right before or during menstruation; strong oral sex; likes clit stimulation only when she is already aroused; likes slow, firm rubbing; thrusting; firm rhythm; rapid penetration with dildos and fingers; strong and fast stimulation when peaking; turned on by fantasies

Preferred positions: all positions except legs up and back

Corn Poppy

Point on the compass: west

Element: earth

Anatomical characteristics: clit and vagina very close to each other, or clit part of the opening; often small hood, or clit peeping out; inner labia small; deep, long cave; tight entry, feels at first penetration like a gate with deep cave behind; G-spot close to vaginal opening (easy orgasm possibilities with fingers, dildos, and vibrators in traditional positions)

Lubrication (wetness): dry

Temperature in cave: hot

Taste: sweet to bitter

Preferences: does not like a lot of "foreplay"; no oral sex; direct stimulation of clitoris can hurt, indirect stimulation through outer labia is better; deep penetration; fast, thrusting penetration with several fingers

Preferred positions: loves all positions, especially legs high behind the head

Noon Flower

Point on the compass: center

Element: mixed qualities from all points of the compass

Anatomical characteristics: clit at the very top; vaginal opening at the very bottom (about three to four fingers distance); consequences: no kinds of visits to the lust cave will indirectly stimulate the clit; small clit with hood, which quickly jumps out when aroused; inner labia narrow; cave moderately deep; G-spot deep and in the back

Lubrication (wetness): moist

Temperature in cave: medium warm

Taste: neutral

Preferences: simultaneous, additional stimulation of pearl when lust tunnel is visited, for example with hand; soft, light pressure on clit; oral sex; sucking; tongue changing from side to side; rubbing

Preferred positions: pillow under small of the back (different angle); close lust-tunnel wandering; kneeling position with straight back; often needs long stimulation to reach orgasm

Many women have recognized and confirmed these descriptions in themselves and others without feeling psychologically and mentally confined, an effect that exclusionary categorizations often have. These descriptions have created an atmosphere of mutual respect, of power through precise knowledge, and of solidarity through sharing this knowledge-power.

The above types are primarily concerned with how to achieve an orgasmic reaction in different women. The Cherokees also explored how to spread orgasmic energy (see Exercise 17, page 102). They suggest the following categories of orgasm, which I have modified and renamed according to my own experiences:

Volcano woman

Explosive like a volcano
Mainly clitorally triggered
With clear boundaries and finely tuned-in energy
A feeling that soon after the spark has been lit the explosion will follow
Multiple climaxes
Like a firework

Snake woman

Internal orgasm that creeps up the spinal cord like a snake
Primarily vaginal
G-spot orgasm
Breathes in strongly; yoni pulls itself in
Body shakes like an earthquake and becomes soft like butter in the sun
Multiple climaxes

Dolphin woman

"Tidal wave"
Implosive beginning, goes in waves from the inside to the outside
One single, deep emotional reaction, often with healing reactions, frequently crying afterwards (reaching the heart level)

Dragon woman

First exuberantly explosive and fiery, then implosive and quieter
Series of mini-orgasms of the clitoral kind, then deeper vaginal orgasm (more inner)
First like shrill, hot wind with sounds, noises, fantasies, images, or salacious words; then quieter and more introverted

Giant woman

Not restricted to the genital area, but rather each body part can be reached with orgasmic sensitivity (in tantra, orgasms are also reached exclusively through breathing and consciousness)
The pulsating of the clit can be part of the orgasm, but the whole body vibrates with pleasure
If this kind experienced, all other kinds can be learned

Our body knows best what kind of orgasm it currently needs. This orgasm often acts as a catalyst for the other kinds, just as the "giant woman" orgasm contains all other variations. It is also the type through which spiritual orgasms (described later in the book) can be reached most easily.

So … what is it like with you?

The Wide Space, Range, and Scope of Ecstasy

What most clearly distinguishes orgasmic sexuality from sensuality, desire, and eroticism is the state of ecstasy. But how can we, as women formed by an ecstasy-hostile society, begin to understand this state? We can approach it by taking little, everyday ecstasies (like the pleasure of the first spoonful of cold, foamy chocolate mousse) seriously, observing them with the same intensity and concentration we normally reserve for the big, celebratory ecstasies (e.g., the love-and-tumble of the first night of a fresh, new love affair).

At this point I don't want to spend time wondering why so many women sacrifice their ecstatic capacity for the everyday, for the "project," or for their conscientious support of "order and discipline." (After all, ecstasy is an anarchic power that often creates disorder.) I would rather use words to describe my experiences and those of other women:

Ecstasy is

the most wonderful way to be outside of yourself and simultaneously to unite with everything, to be one with yourself and the world

the transformation of the physical dimension of love into the spiritual

honoring the universe by pleasurably and respectfully dissolving into it

a little piece of earthly paradise

the greatest anarchic force in our society

losing track of time because of love

The spiritual level of ecstasy, for me and for many women, is an "experienceable" aspect of female existence that is just as much a part of life as the body is, with its needs and reactions. Rather than subscribing to the old patriarchal division of body and soul/spirituality, let us take leave of that view and try a more female, circular, or spiral-shaped way of thinking. Life, desire, and love circulate between material, solid forms of rough energy and delicate, fine forms of spiritual energy, which can become material again. So why exclude a dimension from this spiral? That only interrupts your flow of life energy!

Passionate desire, being in love, and palpable love make it easier to reach this state of ecstasy, but sometimes goodwill, sympathy, a feeling of tender inclination and gentle connection, playfulness, curiosity, and respect for female dignity are enough. "Love alone," however, is not necessarily enough. In my experience with couples who love each other and who come to my therapy sessions because their sexuality has atrophied, it can be helpful not only to work through concrete relationship issues and through individual relationship-building problems, but also to *know more about how to "do it"* so that a partner can come and maybe even keep coming so often that she finally "gets there."

A Short Lesson on the Chakras

It is impossible to discuss tantric sex without an introduction to the chakras. Chakras are rotating energy channels above, around, and within the human body that take care of the organs of their respective regions (see Figure 4 on page 43). The energy generated by each chakra is associated with a particular color. Some of the games and exercises included in this book use the teaching of the chakras to help us guide sexual energy through our bodies (using spiritual images) and to help us understand their different effects within our being.

Since there is an abundance of literature on the subject of chakras (and since it is worthwhile to spend more time looking into this enlightening system), I will offer here only a short list of the characteristics associated with each chakra.

Location means the physical level where the specific energy source of the chakra is located and tangible. Each energy channel supplies specific body parts with life energy; you become more conscious of these body parts when concentrating on this chakra.

Sense means the action and the corresponding sense organ that are most stimulated by the chakra.

Color is the composition of light that is stimulated by the energy of this chakra and what is seen or visualized by most people in relation to this chakra.

Element has to do with the force of nature that is most closely tied to this chakra.

Psychic function refers to the kind of emotionality, the psychic mood that corresponds to the chakra's character.

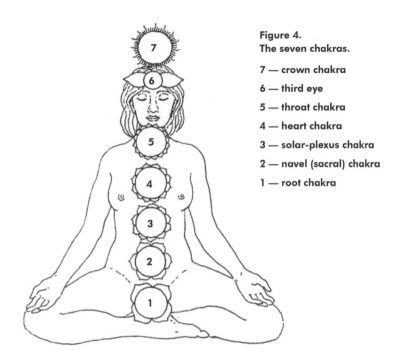

Figure 4.
The seven chakras.

7 — crown chakra

6 — third eye

5 — throat chakra

4 — heart chakra

3 — solar-plexus chakra

2 — navel (sacral) chakra

1 — root chakra

Spiritual theme names the life lesson or life goal that can most easily be reached with the help of this chakra's powers.

The following should form a sufficient basis for the exercises:

1. ROOT CHAKRA
Location: pelvis, perineum
Sense: smell
Energy color: fiery red
Element: earth
Psychic function: will to survive, stability, vitality
Spiritual theme: opening for the healing power of the earth

2. NAVEL (SACRAL) CHAKRA
Location: stomach below the navel, sacrum
Sense: taste
Energy color: orange

Element: water
Psychic function: sexual desire, feelings of being "in the flow"
Spiritual theme: sensuality, desire, vitality

3. SOLAR-PLEXUS CHAKRA
Location: solar plexus, upper stomach, middle back
Sense: sight
Energy color: yellow
Element: fire
Psychic function: self-assuredness, ability to act, power
Spiritual theme: experiencing satisfaction, power, strength

4. HEART CHAKRA
Location: heart, lung
Sense: touch
Energy color: green-pink
Element: air
Psychic function: affection, love, friendliness, joy
Spiritual theme: emanating and receiving love

5. THROAT CHAKRA
Location: throat, neck
Sense: hearing
Energy color: blue
Element: ether
Psychic function: the expression of feelings, creativity, speech
Spiritual theme: freedom of self-expression

6. THIRD EYE
Location: forehead, forming a triangle with the eyebrows
Sense: transcendental
Energy color: violet
Element: no element you can be aware of, but pure, light energy
Psychic function: intuition, extrasensory perception
Spiritual theme: complete recognition of the world

7. CROWN CHAKRA

Location: crown of the head
Sense: feeling of a wide space
Energy color: white-gold
Element: no element, but spacelessness and timelessness
Psychic function: ecstasy, stillness, being
Spiritual theme: oneness with oneself and nature, oneness with the cosmos

These short descriptions and pictures contain many centuries' worth of experiences. However, they are not to be confused with *your* reality! Experiment with them, but rely on your own experiences rather than projecting others' experiences onto yourself. Allow yourself to get to know the depths of your physical self—your living being—better and better!

Sexual Self-Love

All love is self-love. All sexual relationships begin and end with love for oneself. To modify Angelika Aliti's thesis in *Die sinnliche Frau* (The Sensual Woman), we cannot really find outside what we lack inside—if someone cannot feel love, she will most likely not encounter any.

So many women just want to be finally loved but pay little attention to *becoming lovable* themselves. And this ability to be loved begins with the ability to love yourself. A respectful and loving, conscientious and supportive relationship with yourself affects not only your own life, but also your relations with other people and your environment.

One expression of self-love (if not the only one) is sexual self-love, also known as solo sex or autosexuality. Sexual self-love is actually the queen of sexual encounters and relationships, because it can combine a maximum of freedom and autonomy with a maximum of love and honest emotion. This is why it cannot really be replaced by any other form. And this is why some of the activities included in this book are designed for the solo explorer.

Unfortunately, sexual self-love was suppressed for centuries. And although by today's social norms it is now more or less "permitted," it still has a questionable reputation with many, a fear-based reaction connected closely with the devaluation of female sexuality and autonomy. I know many women who ruin their enjoyment of themselves by thinking they have no other options but to pleasure themselves, since no one else is there for them, because they "don't deserve love," or because they see themselves as unattractive in the eyes of others. Or else they are so unattractive in their own eyes, so boring, so unworthy of love, that it never occurs to them to love *themselves;* instead, they just masturbate quickly before going to sleep (even the word seems uninviting to me) in order to release tensions. Or they take no time for sex at all.

Yet *time* is the greatest love-present we can give ourselves in our achievement-oriented society—time without pressure to perform, time to relax, time to listen to yourself, time to spontaneously indulge momentary needs, time to feel and experience. For solo sex I only need to check my own calendar; I can arrange everything however I want, I don't have to consider another person's totally different rhythms, and I am the most important person in this space and time. I can play with my body and my fantasies; I can begin with simple sensuality and develop and experience my body's erotic qualities. I can train my body and my spirit to provide me with orgasms—any orgasms at all, or deeper and bigger ones. I can explore every possible thing and discover what is more and what is less pleasurable for me, and afterward I don't have to wage a battle for the bigger part of the blanket.

I can have the experience of determining and controlling the whole situation myself. I can realize that my newly kindled sexual energy is taking on its own life within me, and that I can only enjoy its strength and breadth if I give up control and give myself over to enjoying the moment. The "reward" is often the state of flow: the happy state of flowing energy and the feeling of being myself, completely at home in the world—an enjoyment that often extends beyond the momentary experience. This is the result of self-love, and at the same time it is a requirement for loving yourself and (out of your inner abundance) the whole world.

One framework for self-love can be a consciously chosen celibate life. In my definition, *celibate* includes all ways of life where sexuality is shared with others rarely, if at all. Instead, it is lived out as self-love, sublimated to life energy, or consciously directed into other channels, such as professional or political engagement, artistic or other creative processes, or spiritually transformed states. Celeste West, in her book *A Lesbian Love Advisor*, describes this state as follows: "Celibacy is the reflective, thought-out confirmation and support of your own self that leads you to direct sexual energy into other channels. It is not to be confused with a coincidental, unwanted state of chastity.... Why set up the requirement that sex must always be directed outward into an orgasm?"

In light of these words, autosexuality is a form of self-love, self-satisfaction, and constructive solitude that can be combined with every type of sexual relationship and preference. This kind of sexuality, present since infancy and particularly repressed in girls, is important not only because it helps them develop their autonomy and female identity along with their corresponding self-confidence, but also because it represents an unceasing (at most, hidden) wellspring of female desire and power. It is not for nothing that our heterocentric culture (and even some lesbian subcultures) sees it as disreputable and is inspired to almost missionary zeal when a woman centers her whole strength in herself rather than letting it flow into the "normal" channels of a relationship. Unfortunately, these "representatives of normalcy" often succeed in turning this state of affairs into a problem, particularly if it has arisen from initially involuntary solitude after a difficult breakup, or if the woman is seen as too attractive not to be "getting some."

In addition, it's becoming very clear to me that even sexuality within a relationship can start out at a much different level of sexual tension—resulting in a much different physical and mental readiness to react—if a woman takes her sexuality seriously enough that she actively integrates it into her everyday life. She gets to know and value herself as a lover, maintains her desire, and does not automatically delegate the responsibility for her satisfaction to her partner. This, in turn, can be very attractive to others.

Below, I've listed some thoughts on revitalizing (or awakening) this aspect of your sexuality. Keep them in mind as you play with the exercises, especially the ones designed for the solo lover:

* All the positive sayings in the world, like "I love myself" or "I think I'm beautiful the way I am," are useless if a woman doesn't already believe them—no matter how big she writes them on the bathroom mirror!

* In my experience, what is much more helpful for a woman who wants to be loving with herself is "pretending." That is, she can try to *act as though* she already loves herself, even if the sentiment behind it is still missing. The result is often that she pampers herself and gradually begins to realize how good it feels. In doing so, she can learn that she is not just an amazed recipient but also a loving giver. Thus, the external role-play gradually becomes a real experience that might just whet the appetite for more self-love.

* Since solo sex, too, is subject to disturbances from that part of a woman's brain where all the memories of unpaid bills, unreturned calls, work stress, irritations, aggravations, and the like compete with one another, it is worthwhile to occupy the brain with *pictures, sounds, and fantasies* (sometimes even set up in advance) so that it can slowly adjust to the idea of desire. For women whose brains are stubbornly occupied with the past and the future rather than the present, it may be necessary to *move, make sounds, and, above all, breathe concentratedly* in order to relax until energy can be made available to build up arousal.

* The most important foundation of well-cultivated autosexual pleasures is the setting aside of restrictive norms and expectations: Solo sex does not need to be perfect, neither from the start nor at all! No one criticizes a woman or devalues her if she doesn't do so herself. Women are often so patient with others—here is an opportunity to practice *patience with yourself,* to encounter yourself with loving understanding as well as patience.

* An important prerequisite is to *give yourself time.* For very busy women like me, this can mean not simply postponing sexual self-love to the weekend and vacations, but scheduling time for it in your routine or in your appointment calendar. You might find this artificial and lacking in spontaneity—it's true—but the alternative can be frustrating: getting nothing at all. Besides, how often do I make plans with others to go out for Chinese food in three weeks, even though when we make the plans I have no idea whether I'll feel like Chinese food that evening, whether I'll be hungry at all, or

whether I will want to meet that particular person at that time. I do it anyway, confirming my grandma's saying: "Your appetite will come when it's time to eat." And when it comes to both pre-planned meals and preplanned sex, your anticipation and conscious inner and outer preparation can contribute to your enjoyment.

✳ For your sexual encounter with yourself to really have a chance to be pleasurable, it is worthwhile to set up *switching-over and transition rituals* (e.g., shaking/dancing/showering off your work-related stress, running once around the block or through the park, making yourself a delightful drink) that will help you to switch over from the energy state of your everyday activities to a relaxed sense of well-being, with the option of pleasurable arousal. Even *relaxation techniques* suited to your own routine—of which there are a great number—can encourage a pleasant "arrival at yourself" (see Exercise 1).

✳ One useful exercise is "Gladdening the heart" (Exercise 17), in which the woman begins stroking herself with fingertips, feathers, or other soft objects and then, step-by-step, arouses herself until the point just *before* climax (or whatever signifies orgasm/ecstasy for her). Then, with a deep breath and a gentle touch of the hands, she draws her energy from the yoni to the level of the heart. Just as she is growing pleasantly relaxed, she begins to arouse herself again. The whole cycle repeats three times in this way; the fourth time, she lets herself fall into her orgasm or finds another way to finish. This is an excellent exercise for creating a gentle kind of self-awareness and for developing a tender relationship with yourself.

✳ If a woman wants to really "blow through" her innermost parts in order to be cleansed and refreshed, she can use the "Fire-breathing orgasm" (Exercise 46), which requires an inner and outer aware-ness of the chakras. As with "Gladdening the heart," the effects of this exercise can be multiplied with practice.

The games and exercises mentioned above, like the others described in this book, are most effective when they are seen as suggestions for helping us call forth our sexual energy. That is, they need not be followed if other wishes make themselves known. Every woman is her own explorer of a realm that belongs only to her, and in which she can do and be whatever she wants.

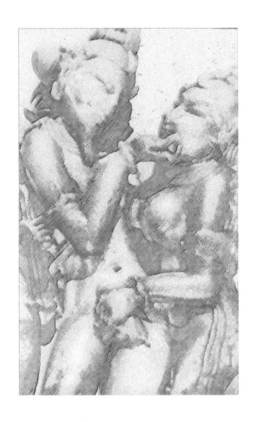

≈ CHAPTER 3 ≈

Enticing Body and Soul into Pleasure

TUNING IN, PLAYING, AND PRACTICING

51

*T*his chapter moves us into the fun stuff: exercises, games, meditations, and rituals, which make up most of the rest of the book. The first part of the chapter offers some guidelines for how to approach the exercises. The later part of the chapter contains what might be thought of as preliminary or preparatory exercises.

In order to make the instructions for the exercises easy to understand, I have generally organized them by theme and goal, time required, necessary preparations, steps to follow, creative ways to deal with stumbling blocks, and possible variations. A few of the exercises include specific music suggestions. For those that don't, some suggestions for music are listed in the Resources section. My recommendations can, of course, be expanded upon or organized differently according to preference. (For example, a woman might find it easier to relax to music with a strong beat, while meditative music might make her slightly nervous.)

As mentioned in the Introduction, since this is a book for women, the exercises don't offer variations involving male body parts, male experiences, or male archetypes. And the pronouns in the exercises usually default to the feminine. Still, if a reader wants to share these love games with a male partner, the two should simply engage their imaginations to come up with creative variations for doing so. Alternatively, using this book in conjunction with a book on tantric sex for mixed-sex partners could create a world of enticing possibilities for a heterosexual couple!

When playing with a partner, practice safer sex. Especially with massages and more intimate games, your responsibility to promote loving contact increases; more importantly, you have a responsibility to avoid leaving any ugly or even life-threatening traces in the form of transmittable diseases (HIV/AIDS, herpes, chlamydia, etc.). This applies especially to contact with mucous membranes, with blood *or any other bodily fluids,* and with abrasions or cuts (even small ones). Inform yourselves about methods of infection, and be open and honest with each other about which safer-sex measures you want or need. If each participant is body- and health-conscious as well as responsible (for themselves and for others), a good foundation will be laid for entering into pleasure-bringing intimacy.

Smart Ways to Manage Distractions

Pleasurable eroticism and sexuality are not miracles; they are the result of a clear decision to take your submission to love, lust, tenderness, and passion more seriously than anything else in the world during the moment of encounter. It follows that there must be intensive internal as well as external preparation of your body and your (possibly stressed-out) soul: preparation of the room, internal and external tuning in to your lover, and, of course, the elimination of as many anaphrodisiacs as possible. (An anaphrodisiac is a hindrance or disturbance that makes it difficult to reach pleasurable heights.) My methods of managing internal disturbances (after taking the utmost care to prevent outside disturbances) are fairly simple:

* *When distracting thoughts come up,* I concentrate even more on my breathing, and I breathe deeper.

* If that doesn't help, I imagine that I am blowing the thoughts out of me when I exhale, thus emptying myself. This gets easier with practice.

* If this is not enough, I imagine a trash can to the left of my love nest and a refrigerator with a big freezer to the right. With a (powerful) exhalation, I toss my "junk thoughts" into the trash can. These are the ones that have been dealt with in therapy but still surface every so often—for example, "I don't deserve to be desired this much!" I imagine placing the thoughts that are definitely important but unnecessary at the moment (e.g., "Hey, I could record this feeling in the form of a poem!") in the freezer, promising myself I will get them out tomorrow and give them the attention they deserve. Then I concentrate on the most pleasurable part of my body or on two loving eyes or on my breath again.

* Sometimes, with persistently interfering thoughts, a disciplined "Not now!" followed by concentration on my internal breathing helps.

* *With distracting physical sensations* (like ticklishness or pain), a short communiqué—a request to be touched elsewhere or to

change positions—usually helps. So does deeper breathing. (I'll put off the psychological analysis of ticklishness as a possible inner defense mechanism for later.)

* If the sensations persist, taking a short break, concentrating on the feelings triggered by the sexual encounter, or choosing a new way to access my body often helps.

* *With distracting feelings or thoughts about my partner(s)*, it usually helps to express the feeling in a brief, noninsulting way. (Insults usually set off a destructive spiral.) It may also work to use some of the above ideas that apply to interfering thoughts in general.

* Sometimes there's no way to avoid a full-blown argument with your partner; still, it's usually possible to create a distraction-free island where unresolved relationship problems, for example, have no business intruding. The advanced exercises aim to let you be undisturbed by relationship problems, instead disturbing *them* with your increased desire.

Appreciating Apathy

Sometimes, during a sensual interlude, a lack of sexual desire will crop up seemingly out of nowhere. Accepting the challenge of changing this apathy back into eroticism is an important basis of the womanly art of love. Doing so means smart management of suddenly appearing anaphrodisiacs, such as stress and a lack of desire.

If, in your encounter with your beloved, desire suddenly turns into apathy, there are several possible ways to create a change. Usually, one or two of the following steps will prove to be enough:

* Name your feelings of apathy and express them with your entire body.

* Exaggerate your apathy until it becomes clear on the relationship level—until both parties understand its meaning and its function in your momentary encounter or in the relationship.

* Ask each other (rather than immediately assuming you know the

answer) whether a secret, half-conscious *yes* is hiding behind the *no* of apathy. If this is the case, find out what you can say yes to.

✳ Try to find other ways to resolve your expressions of apathy. If, for example, you feel like setting limits on your beloved's enormous expectations for sex between the two of you, instead free yourselves by engaging in a wild romp in which those fastidious demands simply fade away with the gasping of a woman who is doubled over in laughter.

✳ Come to a conscious decision that you will give desire and its awakening more space, inside and out, than you give to your preoccupation with creating or maintaining apathy.

✳ Accept your apathetic reaction as an individual expression of life—one that does not need to be overinterpreted right now but is allowed to exist as a state of its own.

Just as light enlightens the darkness, desire can embrace and transform apathy. This may sound hard or even impossible, but in my experience the distance from apathy to desire is sometimes much smaller than I expect! It's more a question of your internal attitude than of external circumstances. This means it takes a conscious decision not to let desire be ruined by apathy. But it also means it is up to you to *disturb disturbances with desire,* to shake them up and transform them (into an energetic, aggressive pillow fight, for example).

Six Keys to the Gates of Physical Pleasure

Together, the following six practices are a highly recommended preexercise for all the other games and exercises. They can be practiced in every possible life situation, even nonsexual ones.

1. Deep breathing: This means consciously and constantly raising the volume of your breathing in order to better perceive and express your feelings. In this concentration on deep breathing lies the secret to many methods that can increase your capabilities for love and ecstasy. It allows us to turn away from the many ideas, judgments, evaluations, memories, and plans for the future that lie in the backs of our minds, and to turn instead toward our bodies and the current encounter. Caution is advised here if a woman tends to hyperventilate (make sure to exhale completely!), but most of us tend to breathe shallowly, so our stomach and chest areas could do with more oxygen anyway. When we inhale more oxygen than our body needs, we create an energy field around ourselves that can nourish and protect us.

2. *Spontaneous movement:* This is less about targeted movements than it is about the ability to give in to strong as well as subtle impulses to move your body, to "let yourself be moved by your inner (e)motion." It is also about the ability to perceive the often very delicate movements of your internal organs, muscles, and circulation, and to give yourself over to these perceptions. If my body is flexible, I am more flexible with others, and I can express my feelings even without many words.

3. *Sounds and tones:* Since many women—if they didn't happen to be raised "like boys"—have learned to be proper and quiet, and never crooked, shrill, or loud, it often takes a long time for us to recognize our own sounds of pleasure or displeasure, let alone to express them. These sounds and tones, however, are especially good for transporting the energy of our feelings "to the outside," so that refusing to "sound off" often gives an imprecise indication of our feelings. Besides, when we make a variety of noises, it's much easier for our lovers to understand us. And hearing our own sounds can strengthen our own sensations as well.

It's a good preliminary exercise (at least in private) to accompany *every* movement with sounds—groaning, moaning, growling, giggling, humming, singing, etc. This not only makes the emotional quality of movement clear, but it also often makes movement itself easier.

4. *Concentration and consciousness:* As we know, in our everyday lives there are countless ways to divert our attention from ourselves and from close contact with others. Cultivated sexuality is less

about figuring out techniques than it is about having a loving, concentrated awareness of our feelings and encounters. This relaxed concentration is what can make every instant a conscious and special experience.

A good way to practice concentrating on the famous "here and now" is to imagine that with one deep breath you are pulling all your experiences of attraction, love, and ecstasy into your heart and concentrating them there in your own center of love. (One particular method for bundling and then distributing sexual energy is the "big draw"; see within Exercise 47, page 195.) We let all other experiences, memories, or plans for the future float away like clouds in the sky, or else we imagine releasing them when we exhale. If they persist in pushing to the forefront of our consciousness, we do not fight them (that would be giving too much energy to useless things!); instead, we symbolically put them into that imaginary refrigerator next to the love nest, where they will stay "fresh" and can be taken out again the next day (if, for example, I suddenly have a great idea for redecorating the bedroom).

5. *Playing in the moment:* Being happy in the moment is usually less about purpose-driven and goal-oriented action than about playing out of a pure "love of joy" or the ability to "let your soul dangle" and give yourself over to the sensations of the moment. The further development of female sexuality is not the result of behavioral training, but rather of the courage to take risks; it comes from trial and error (sometimes a lot of error), from a sense of humor, and from the combining of childish curiosity with adult longings. Through playful, experimental trying we can have new experiences that do not necessarily have to be "perfect" or complete. This makes it easier to take the performance pressure out of sex and to *be* together without trying to reach a goal (e.g., multiple orgasms).

6. *Practice and habit:* Even if wonderful sexual experiences can never be repeated exactly, we can, with regular practice, prepare our

bodies (i.e., the pelvic muscles, the heart muscles, and the circulation), our souls (i.e., the ability to open ourselves to the right person in the right moment and then to close again), our minds (i.e., understanding our own possibilities and boundaries), and our spirituality (i.e., the perception of our connection with nature and our oneness with the world), and make them open to pleasure and joy. If we make practice a habit by integrating it into our daily routine, ecstasy will no longer be a rare weekend and holiday feeling, but can even cast doing the dishes in a new light.

Magic Pleasure Potions: Aphrodisiacs

Aphrodite, the goddess of love and desire in the patriarchal Greek pantheon, developed an enormous amount of creativity in order to promote sensuality, eroticism, desire, and passion among the gods and human beings. She desired these things herself, so all the means to these ends are called *aphrodisiacs*. The goddess, born of foam, understood (as did Sappho) how to entice the senses with simple methods, thereby training the body's perception and preparing it for sexual pleasures. The most effective aphrodisiacs are, of course, loving and being in love, passion, and tenderness, followed closely by honest compliments, flowers, sensual music, and an appropriate ambiance. Why not add a little extra spice to this setup?

In cultures where sensuality and sexuality have always been valued more highly than in the West—for example, in the Egypt or India of old—aphrodisiacs were researched as a matter of course and used creatively. Worldwide, there are about a thousand plants and innumerable animal products that are known for their aphrodisiac effects. Some of these are too foreign for our Western palates or are regulated by the FDA or have excessive side effects. But my experiences with, for example, the "fire drink" (a brew of twelve different aphrodisiacs, mixed under a full moon) and other desire-enhancing fruit and vegetable drinks have been so positive that I want to give you at least a few suggestions. Beyond these, I refer you to the many books on this topic.

In terms of food, it's important that it not be too rich, too heavy, or too sour, since that would keep the blood occupied with the digestive organs and prevent it from providing oxygen to the body's erotic parts, such

as the yoni, nipples, or even knee joints. The result can be a pleasant lazi-
ness that causes the longed-for evening to end happily in front of the TV
or that turns your breathing during cuddling into snoring. That's fine, of
course, as long as you both want it that way.

Neither the famous oysters nor the classic champagne can fan a flame
where nothing exists; however, even tiny flames can be tended! Aphrodisiac
foods, herbs, and scents have the inestimable advantage of stimulating all
the senses and leading even hard-boiled individuals into a state of sensuality and of giving in to the moment!

The following is a small assortment of aphrodisiacs that are not drugs
(according to our cultural definition), have no significant side effects, and
are easy to come by or make:

Herbs and spices: basil, cardamom, chili, cinnamon, cloves, ginger,
lovage, mint, muscat, oregano, parsley, pepper, rosemary, and saffron

Vegetarian options: almonds, apples, apricots, avocados, carrots, cel-
ery, chocolate, fennel, figs, grapes, mangoes, mushrooms, nuts,
peaches, plums, pomegranates, quinces, strawberries, and tomatoes

Seafood: eel, mussels, oysters, salmon, shrimp, and snails

Drinks: drinks containing any of the fruits listed under "vegetarian
options," mixed with sparkling, low-sodium mineral water or
sparkling wine and spiced with a touch of pepper and/or honey
and/or cinnamon; coffee with cardamom; tea with ginger, cardamom, cloves, black pepper, and cinnamon

Scents: above all, your body's own scents, especially fresh perspiration
or spicy yoni-scent; plant scents: amber, carnation, hyacinth, (white)
musk, narcissus, orange blossom, and rose; scented oils (be careful
about the ingredients!), including cinnamon, geranium, jasmine, mus-
catel, sage, neroli, rose (preferably Moroccan; its scent has a special
depth and is not as room-filling as the scent of the Bulgarian rose),
sandalwood, vanilla, and ylang-ylang

This small assortment probably includes things that could "set you
off" right away as well as some you don't like at all. Try out the ones you

like and the ones you know your partner at least doesn't dislike. Let yourself be inspired by creative mixtures and sensual decorations! For more information, see the Resources section.

Naturally, all these wonderful scents, foods, and drinks have the greatest effect when given in conjunction with compliments. Even if I only have plain water available, I can administer it to my beloved sip by sip and compliment by compliment; that is, I can whisper a compliment into her ear and then give her a sip to drink, so that she can't contradict me! If she wants to return the compliment right away instead of drawing it into herself first, I can stop her mouth with another sip. This little manipulation is usually accepted without any serious protest....

A less beloved, but highly effective, aphrodisiac is temporary renouncement of your lover. Many long-distance lovers and partners of very busy individuals are familiar with this as an involuntary act that, along with frustration and anger, usually increases longing. Even more effective, however, is a temporary, *voluntary* renunciation. In addition to longing, voluntarily imposing time away from each other offers anticipation—assuming the separation doesn't last too long and that upon being reunited both people don't throw themselves at each other as if starving. Rather, take cautious steps to allow intimacy.

A simple little aphrodisiac involves spoiling your body while occupying your brain—for example, with "spiced-up" reading. If you want to put your lover in a sexual mood, but she or he would rather read in bed, you not only "allow" your partner to do that, you even order her or him, in as strict a tone as possible, to keep reading no matter what happens. Then you slowly and steadily begin to stroke, kiss, lick, or nibble your partner's body from head to toe. If your beloved tries to react, either positively or negatively, order her or him even more strictly to please concentrate on reading. When your lover is gasping for air and wants to throw the book aside, order her or him to read aloud to you, keeping her or his hands on the book. Only when your lover's body is already "there" do you allow her or him to come under your fiery caresses.

Yes, these pleasure potions are terrific, but what if the stumbling blocks in someone who is plagued by norms and stress are stronger than chocolate? My suggestion is to recognize them, understand them, appreciate them, and *actively* say good-bye to them so that you, as a contemporary woman, can take over the responsibility for the present and try something new.

How can you achieve this? With the power of the mind and your energetic will! (I know it very well myself: the old thinking that my fears from the past might outweigh my lust for ecstatic sexual play with others in the present. A wise tantra teacher once told me, "Do you know, Christa, why bumblebees can fly, even though their large bodies in relation to their small wings make it almost physically impossible? Because they wanted it at that moment and they summoned up all their energies to take off!" I am not a biologist, but the bumblebee identity that I have since adopted enables me to do all kinds of "impossible" things.)

In this sense, the exercises included in this chapter serve as preparation—first for the mind and the spirit, and then for the body—so you can become able to perceive, allow, and express more and more pleasure. From the following exercises, choose the ones that promise the most relief. Choose the ones that make you curious and the ones that promise fun for your current mood. In other words, it's not about wading through the exercises in the order in which they appear, but rather about a spontaneous selection, with the goal that the exercises described later can take their full effect and continue to have a pleasurable effect long afterward.

If, on the other hand, you and the person you are in love with have the impression that you are wonderfully open and able to flow, don't linger on the preliminaries. Start with even more enjoyable forms of foreplay, such as the breast massage exercises in Chapter 7....

🐝 Exercise 1: Shaking off the outside world and arriving in your own body

Many women have trouble letting themselves fall into sexual desire and ecstasy because evenings and even weekends are times when they are filled with ideas, plans, memories, and stresses; that is, their heads are full. The female body, too, which often must spend hours in front of the computer or running back and forth from the kindergarten to the grocery store to the dry cleaner, is full of tension. It's no wonder that some women can no longer imagine having time for pleasure after work.

One way to rid yourself of some everyday stress and gradually switch over to other forms of energy is to engage in transitional or switching-over rituals. Most women have these rituals, even if they wouldn't call them that; examples might include taking a shower and changing clothes after work, running around the block with the dog, or drinking a good cup of tea in peace. The movement meditations that follow are intended especially for switching over from everyday stress to evening or weekend relaxation.

GOAL

This action meditation helps shake off everyday stress and helps you prepare to create inner stillness, not by forbidding the use of speech, but by allowing it and even powerfully exaggerating it.

TIME AND EXTERNAL PREPARATIONS

About sixty minutes in four phases; a room where you can be undisturbed (of course, this holds true for almost every exercise).

STEP BY STEP

I. *Shaking:* In a loose stance, stand up straight and with your feet hip-width apart and begin to move your knees forward and back, easily and quickly, so that a shaking motion develops, spreading throughout your whole body. (If you are familiar with kundalini meditation, you can use that kind of shaking.) Meanwhile, imagine that you are shaking out all your stress, all your gummed-up and tense muscles, all your stiffness and uncomfortable postures. Shake off your spiritual and mental stress, too. While doing so, breathe with your mouth open. Your relief will be greater if, while you're shaking, you let not only sweat come out of your pores but also sounds come out of your mouth. Since you have a quarter of an hour to shake every shakable part, you can also go through the various parts of your body and focus on individual parts by themselves (arms, legs, hips, etc.). And if a specific remark from your boss or a colleague is still sitting "in your bones," imagine that you are shaking it out of yourself; if you notice you are upset about something, stomp it into the floor.

2. *Babbling:* Next, sit down and utter nonsense syllables for fifteen minutes. Here is your opportunity to bring into being, with sounds, all those things you've never expressed in words or any new kinds of feelings that come up. Support these sounds with strong gestures, by expressing what you have to say with your whole body; go ahead and exaggerate. Give yourself permission to be a little "hysterical"!

3. *Sinking down:* Now lie down on a soft surface and investigate any changes that might have taken place in your feelings and perceptions now that you've been able to release at least some of your inner tension. Let yourself become calmer with each breath, emphasize your exhalations, and imagine that with every exhalation you are sinking deeper and deeper into the mattress or blanket under you. Imagine that you are getting flatter and flatter, until finally you are lying there like a little flounder. Then concentrate on your knees, which are probably not lying completely flat. Imagine that your tendons are growing more flexible with every breath, so that your knee joints gradually sink down lower and lower.

   After a while, move your attention to your sacrum, or lower back; you may find that you have an arch that reaches up toward your middle back. If this arch hurts too much, you can bend your knees and place the soles of your feet on the ground every so often in order to change your back position. Otherwise, imagine that this body part, too, is sinking lower and lower into the mat with every exhalation. Sometimes it's helpful to visualize a sail that billows out as you inhale and then sinks lower every time you breathe out.

   After a little while, transfer your attention to your neck and throat; imagine that your neck is moving lower and lower as you breathe out and that the nape of your neck is gently sinking in. Then breathe deeply through the length of your body, and imagine that your entire body is sinking further into the mat and that you are being carried by the mat.

4. *Dreaming:* Become aware of the stillness inside you that underlies the sounds, tones, and movements of the earlier steps. Even if all kinds of thoughts come to the surface, let them come out of you like little air bubbles when you breathe out and keep concentrating on the feeling of being carried. Let yourself dream. Dream yourself into a landscape (or a room) where you can relax, where you feel comfortable and can be happily alone with yourself. Take about fifteen minutes for this phase and allow yourself to linger in your dreamworld. If you are measuring the time yourself, don't call yourself back to reality with a loud alarm clock; find other ways to mark the time or even to stretch it out.

CREATIVE WAYS TO DEAL WITH STUMBLING BLOCKS

The tendency to break off early, especially in the "babbling phase," with the thought "Okay, that's enough!" or "I'm just repeating myself!" or "I don't have anything else to express!" is totally normal at the beginning. In order to keep from getting stuck in this way, it's worth resolving, before you start the meditation, to complete the forty-five minutes of shaking, babbling, and meditating no matter what. This will allow you to reach a deeper level of relaxation than if you were to babble for only five minutes. It may be that you feel overwhelmed by distracting thoughts in steps 2 through 4. If so, you should try to concentrate on your breathing or your respective body parts; during the dream phase, try to transform any stressful thoughts so that they fit into a pleasant dreamscape.

VARIATIONS AND SUGGESTIONS

During the "babbling phase," try having a medium-firm pillow in front of you so you can punch it without hurting yourself if you happen to get angry.

🕊 Exercise 2: In the lap of Mother Earth

If we are well rooted in the earth, we can grow, stretch out, bloom. Being connected to the earth gives our spiritual development a nourishing bed and helps keep us from "lifting off" or losing contact with our own bodies. Besides, we need a strong but flexible trunk that will keep us from falling over or being uprooted by sudden storms; this allows us to give in to various other forces.

Some women are afraid of losing themselves in dreams. Some are especially afraid of losing their boundaries, their selves, during sex, because they might be swept away by too much passion. This can happen easily if a woman is not comfortable with herself and doesn't feel well grounded.

You can practice this grounding exercise before and after every energizing exercise so that you will feel safely rooted and can pass on all your excess energy to the earth.

GOAL

You can emphasize your connection to the earth as a preparation and wind-down of your body and soul for almost all of the following exercises, games, rituals, and meditations; doing so will prevent you from "lifting off" in all directions and will help you keep both feet on the ground.

TIME AND EXTERNAL PREPARATIONS

Fifteen minutes before and after other exercises. It is easier if you record the instructions on a cassette tape ahead of time, or have someone read them to you.

STEP BY STEP

* Stand up straight with your feet hip-width apart, knees loose. Loosen any restrictive clothing and breathe deeply.

* Stomp your feet a couple of times until you have the feeling that your soles are well connected with the ground.

* Bend your knees a little more and relax your jaw. Breathe deeply through the length of your body.

* Now lay a hand on your yoni or (with shorter breaths) on your mons veneris; imagine breathing out into your hand until your yoni is full of breath, well circulated and alive. Now release your hand and continue to breathe into your yoni.

* Imagine that roots are growing out of your yoni. They get longer with every breath and grow deeper and deeper into the earth. Your yoni-roots find their way through many layers of sand, clay, and

stone to the middle of the planet, the lap of Mother Earth. There, where the fiery red magma flows, your roots dive into her heat.

✳ Everything—all the tensions and unnecessary thoughts that you put into your exhalation and send down into her lap—is accepted and transformed there into pure energy. The fiery lap of the earth knows no difference between "good" and "bad" energy. You can give it everything, and likewise you can take in as much energy as you need with each breath. The energy you take in cools off on its journey back up through the layers of sand and rock, so that its scorching heat becomes comforting warmth. Warm yourself with this breath. Pull the energy up so forcefully that it flows warmly through your yoni, your belly, your heart, your throat, and your head, and let it wash out any remaining waste and stumbling blocks when you breathe out.

✳ When your whole "trunk" feels somewhat cleaner and more relieved, lift your arms like the crown of a tree growing out of the trunk. Breathe high into your fingertips and stretch them as though you are trying to touch the sky.

✳ Let your breath fill the whole length of your body—from your roots, resting securely in the lap of Mother Earth, to your crown, reaching into the sky. Like a tree, you can sway gently in the wind while remaining firmly anchored in the ground.

✳ Now let your arms sink down slowly, and cross your hands on your chest over your heart. Breathe deeply into the heart space under your hands and remind yourself that the heart represents the midpoint between above and below, between roots and crown. Make an inner picture for yourself of how your breathing energy and the life energy of your roots and crown meet here and fuse together.

✳ Once your heart is loaded up with breathing energy, open your arms and imagine whom you would like to invite into your heart space or what areas and levels you would like to expand into.

* Finally, stand calmly for a moment and let this experience resonate in your innermost being.

CREATIVE WAYS TO DEAL WITH STUMBLING BLOCKS
If you are afraid that you and your roots will be swallowed by a giant vulva, picture the nourishing and giving quality of the female lap. If other threatening or destructive fantasies come up, take them as a sign of the unconscious destructiveness within you; don't give them a moment's thought, and instead move on to more pleasant images. The images you choose can be different from mine—after all, it's *your* grounding exercise!

VARIATIONS AND SUGGESTIONS
This exercise could be even more effective if performed on the soft ground of a forest or meadow rather than behind closed doors.

🕊 Exercise 3: Smiling inside

This is a Taoist meditation practice that improves our consciousness, self-acceptance, circulation, and the free flow of energy in every organ and its respective chakra. Here we restrict our concentration to the sexual organs.

GOAL
The conscious and loving acceptance of each and every body part.

TIME AND EXTERNAL PREPARATIONS
Two minutes and a quiet room are all you need to feel a positive effect. With a little more time, more organs or body parts could be included.

STEP BY STEP
* Breathe deeply in and out a couple of times.

* Then concentrate on your breasts, for example, or your yoni, and consciously let your breath flow through this particular part of your body.

* Now move first the right, then the left corner of your mouth toward your ears. Yes, exactly: Smile silently at yourself and at your breasts or your yoni!

* While smiling, give them the most tender attention possible. In doing so, give yourself as a woman gentle, tender, and calm attention—the kind you might usually give to a lover. You are your own most significant and most faithful lover!

CREATIVE WAYS TO DEAL WITH STUMBLING BLOCKS

Of course, it's possible to fall into a (self-)critical observation of your breasts, for example, and find fault with them. If this occurs, remember: Every problem that arises is an opportunity for further development—it's just an opportunity in work clothes.

In order to keep from getting stuck in familiar, old patterns of belittling yourself, try to concentrate particularly on the flow of your breath *inside* or imagine that you are giving thanks for your breasts and honoring their lifelong being-there-for-you.

If this doesn't help, you can imagine that a lover or even an enlightened being is looking at them with great joy and stroking them with a gentle smile.

If the thought of being your own best lover threatens to depress you (as in: "No one else loves me anyway"), then try even a crooked grin. Keep it up until your mood changes.

VARIATIONS AND SUGGESTIONS

If you have lost tissue from one or both breasts, for example to cancer, hold and touch the scar tissue especially gently with your hands. If tears of grief or pain come, let them fall onto your breasts and see if you can stroke them from inside using a survivor's knowing, benevolent smile.

In a more advanced variation of the exercise, let your inner smile move to the third eye and then let it flow from there to your breasts or yoni.

A further variation has to do with the thought that your inner smile is flowing through the crown chakra like a little fountain, into the higher levels of the aura, in order to rain down on your breasts in many small droplets of joy.

🐫 Exercise 4: Camel ride in your own bedroom

Some readers have probably ridden a camel before and are thus familiar with that rocking motion in the loins. After the first feelings of strangeness have passed, the ride grows more enjoyable as the rider lets her lower back become more flexible, and the more she passively *allows* her movements to happen rather than performing them actively. We don't have to travel to distant lands to experience this sensation. We can enjoy the "pelvic swing," familiar to many, under a summer sun or at home in a cozy, warm room filled with the sounds of sensual music.

GOAL

Allowing the pelvis to grow softer and more receptive, and letting erotic-sexual energy flow horizontally as well as vertically (see also "Full-moon meditation," Exercise 53).

TIME AND EXTERNAL PREPARATIONS

Twenty minutes and a meditation pillow.

STEP BY STEP

* Sit up straight so that you can feel your sit bones. Breathing in, let your pelvis swing backward while your rib cage passively bends forward a little. Breathing out, your pelvis will swing gently forward while your upper body swings slightly back. This will help you begin a gentle wave motion. While doing this, imagine that, when inhaling, you are drawing all your energy in and back; when exhaling, you are pushing it forward with opened labia.

* Play with different rocking motions—bigger and smaller, faster and slower.

* Finally, let the motions grow so small that they are no longer perceptible from the outside; however, the inner wave motion continues within you.

CREATIVE WAYS TO DEAL WITH STUMBLING BLOCKS

If you are trying to do it "right" no matter what, you may be straining your pelvis too much. As a result, your movements will become stiff and laborious. Instead, make it easy for yourself and rock yourself until you feel like you could keep rocking back and forth forever.

VARIATIONS AND SUGGESTIONS

If you are sitting across from a partner during this exercise, keep your eyes closed at first so that you can start with yourself. Then you can imagine that you are drawing sexual energy from your partner, and giving it back to that person through your labia when you exhale. Afterward, open your eyes and move your eyelids in concert with your labia. If an erotic charge happens to flow between your pupils, allow this flow and observe it with your inner eye.

✍ Exercise 5: The power of the tigress

The fiery energy of our sexual ecstasy can be fanned to a greater flame much more easily when our bodies are more receptive and able to oscillate. Part of this is due to the famed PC muscle. One of its layers encircles the pearl of the clitoris and the anus in a figure eight, crossing over the perineum (see Figure 3, page 31). It is the part of the pelvic musculature that is most responsible for orgasmic movement, and its flexibility and circulation greatly influence the depth, length, intensity, and number of our orgasms. If we exercise it a little by stretching and contracting it, we can increase the power of our desire on the physical level as well.

GOAL

Improving the circulation and range of motion of the entire pelvic floor, whereby the clitoris, vagina, anus, and perineum are energized, too. As a result, our orgasms can become more frequent, deeper, stronger, and longer.

TIME AND EXTERNAL PREPARATIONS

A few minutes a day are all you need for short exercise units. Since this exercise plays out internally, you can do this exercise almost any time—at boring conferences, at red lights, in the bus, and on the train. It's best not to wait until you feel like doing this little exercise; just do it whenever you happen to think about it.

STEP BY STEP

* In order to identify the muscle, try to interrupt the flow of urine when you're peeing. If it works, you've found your lowermost pleasure muscle.

* In order to exercise it, it's best to start by yourself: Sit down comfortably and lay your hand on your perineum—the crossing point of this lasso-like figure-eight muscle. Then imagine that you're waiting in a long line of women who all have to go to the bathroom. In order to "stay dry," you pull the muscle together and upward. Then imagine that you're finally sitting on the toilet and can relax everything and let go. You can repeat this cycle of contracting and letting go up to thirty times (no more than that when you start, or you might get a little PC-muscle cramp).

* Next, imagine that your PC muscle is dancing a three-beat waltz: When you breathe in, you can contract, release, contract, or vice versa. It doesn't matter whether you choose a quick Viennese waltz or a slow one; just play a little with this balance between tension and relaxation.

* Now imagine that you are a little girl in a colorful meadow. Whenever you see a flower you like, you squat directly over it and imagine that you are using your PC muscle to pick it and draw it upward into your belly. This emphasizes the upward motion when you contract. After you've picked it, let go again until you have found the next pretty flower. Slowly, a whole bouquet—which you'd like to give to some nice person—is collecting in your belly. So you inhale deeply, and with the next breath out you push the bouquet out of you, so that it falls through your vagina into the grass. This image, or one of your own, can help you practice the difference between pulling in and pressing out.

* Relax for a moment and sit down with your back leaning against something, again with your hand on your perineum. This time you don't have to change or contract anything actively; just observe what happens when you (a) cough, (b) sneeze, (c) laugh.

* Then, lying down on your back, stretch out, and use your fingertips to tap on your perineum. Play a little more with pulling the PC muscle in and pressing out, and imagine that the little movement of the muscle has taken over the whole length of your body and is making it permeable.

✳ If it makes the game easier, you can also tense the PC muscle—briefly and powerfully—in moments of great arousal. This will bring your sexual energy from the bottom to the top in one big rush.

CREATIVE WAYS TO DEAL WITH STUMBLING BLOCKS
You may be frustrated because you can't feel everything right away. This is normal when a muscle and the nerves that go with it are still in hibernation. Take your time and practice: It won't fail to have an effect, and there's always a light at the end of the tunnel!

For some women, a love of details helps them recognize and honor even minimal changes (which are what count here) in themselves.

VARIATIONS AND SUGGESTIONS
The exercises with coughing, sneezing, and laughing in particular are more fun with two people sitting across from each other.

If you have a partner for this, you can ask that person to place a hand on your perineum so you can devote yourself to your sensations without straining your arm muscles.

🗡 Exercise 6: The wild fire-woman's meditation

Not only the outer but also the inner flame needs to be fanned, strengthened, and expressed—and the more your body is energetically charged, the more clearly and strongly you will experience all the feelings that are within you. For maximum strength of feelings, the following holds true: The more you breathe and make sounds and move around, the more charged up you will be. Just try it!

GOAL
Discovering, increasing, and expressing your inner fire, and recognizing it in its various forms.

TIME AND EXTERNAL PREPARATIONS
About an hour, in four phases.

STEP BY STEP

1. *Shaking:* For fifteen minutes, shake every part of yourself. Concentrate on leaving your jaw loose, and try out various rhythms, strengths, and combinations of shaking (see Exercise I).

2. *Fire dance:* In the next fifteen minutes, move with drum music and follow your body's impulses. Pay attention to any and all movement impulses and give in to them; make them stronger and express them, let them spread out. These can be stomping, hopping, dancing, or shaking movements that you can emphasize by making sounds.

3. *Swinging:* Lie down and bend your legs; place your feet hip-width apart, and lay your right hand on your yoni and the left one on your heart chakra. Now let your attention and your breath flow between your yoni and your heart for fifteen minutes. This flow of breath between your lap and your heart is like the breath of Mother Earth, which flows calmly and steadily, and occasionally includes the fiery power of volcanoes. Afterward, slowly open your knees as you inhale, and slowly close them again as you exhale. Imagine that you are resting on Mother Earth like a firebird that is moving its wings in preparation for swooping up into the air and that then lands and flys again.

4. *Landing:* This quarter of an hour allows you to increase and spread the relaxation you are feeling. You can stretch out your legs and relax, cover yourself, and investigate your breathing. Your hands can lie loosely on your yoni and your heart, or not; what is important is being aware of your breathing, your pulse, your warmth, and your entire body, which right now may feel more like a bed of calm embers than the smoldering flames of the earlier phases. Allow yourself to experience all your feelings and sensations as they are right now—to feel yourself as you happen to be at this moment.

CREATIVE WAYS TO DEAL WITH STUMBLING BLOCKS

Some women are surprised by how exhausted they get in the first two phases or by how restless they feel in the next two. If you become exhausted quickly, make your movements smaller but do not stop moving; if you feel restless, it sometimes helps to deepen your breathing and to concentrate on the parts of your body that you are most conscious of at the moment.

VARIATIONS AND SUGGESTIONS

In the second phase, it helps to activate your inner fire-woman by imagining that you are a fire or a dancing flame; in doing so, you can experience more of the aggressive, destructive power of fire or its erotic sexual aspect in your imagination and your movements.

🐉 Exercise 7: The dancing dragon-woman

(This meditation was suggested by Maria Kennerknecht and, like almost all of the meditations, was developed further through mutual practice.)

Even if dragons have allegedly long been extinct, they do exist—in the form of wild women who breathe fire, fly (internally), move freely about the earth, and can take on all kinds of characteristics.

GOAL

To dance through the various elements as a dragon-woman, thereby acknowledging and expressing the special qualities in yourself.

TIME AND EXTERNAL PREPARATIONS

Sixty minutes; a big room where you can also be loud.

STEP BY STEP

Your movements can be gentle or wild, small or large. They should always emanate from your pelvis, so that they flow outward from the inside. Accompany your dance with gestures, humming, and singing so you can physically experience the elements' differing qualities and the power they hold. This helps make you more aware of them, and you will notice that you yourself produce and strengthen these different energy qualities and the moods that accompany them.

This movement meditation has six phases of ten minutes each:

1. *Singing the big "U" (oooh) and moving in your body until you become a dragon-woman.* Stand upright, your feet hip-width apart, your knees loosely bent. Straighten your spine so that your head is being carried upright. Let your shoulders sink down, and loosen your chin and jaw. Breathe deeply in and out a couple of times. Then breathe even more deeply into your belly and pelvis. Imagine that there is a big letter U in the middle of your pelvis. The U wants to be expressed, and you begin to sound it, singing or calling to it. Then imagine that the U begins to move, rolling around in your pelvis while you continue to bring it into the room through your throat. Its movements become more varied: It can circle, tumble, roll, bump, or rock itself, which causes different sounds to emanate from your throat. The U is a deep and a curious belly-letter. It wants to explore your whole pelvis. Let it have its fun. Then, in the deepest recesses of your pelvic floor, the U discovers a dragon-woman. Let her figure grow clearer inside you. As you keep doing this, you gradually *become* a restless dragon-woman, in whom the sounds and movements are one.

2. *Dancing the element of water until you become a sea serpent.* The figure of the dragon-woman grows more and more lively. She wriggles, raises her head, and reveals herself to be a supple, shimmering, magical dragoness. She moves flowingly, and you follow her movements. She dives into the water element and becomes a sea serpent. As a sea serpent, she glides through the waves and currents of the water. As a sea serpent, turn and rock your pelvis, wriggle your arms, bend and turn your torso. Your steps are soft, and your movements grow softer, rounder, and more flowing. Sometimes they are small, sometimes large, sometimes gentle, sometimes wild—whatever pleases the sea serpent within you. Give yourself over to the ocean of your feelings. Let yourself drift gradually to the shore.

3. *Dancing the element of earth until you become a gigantic dragoness.* When you are on the shore and feel solid ground

beneath your feet, you turn back into the dragoness who is certain of her contact with the earth. Take a walk around your territory, decisively. Walk with broad strides, powerfully, but without locking your knees. With every step, your feet are connected to the earth. Your gait is clear and makes you an impressive figure. Your movements still emanate from your pelvis, which is comfortably rocking and circling. Doing this, you take in your space—conscious of yourself—and find, through your connection to the earth, your connection to your ancestors.

4. *Dancing the element of fire until you become a fire-breathing, erotic dragoness.* From the security of her contact with the earth, the dragon-woman now fans her inner flame. As a fire-dragoness, she sprays, hisses, and spits with a lust for life—or with rage, if something displeases her. She sprays pure fire from her mouth, nose, and eyes. Her fiery temperament shows itself through quick, sassy hip movements and a proud straightening of the upper body and head. She stretches luxuriously and shakes off little sparks and flames. You become, more and more, a spark-spraying being of energy. As a dragon-woman, you are seduction personified: erotic from head to toe, alluring, passionate, simply irresistible. You put all your energy into your fire dance.

5. *Dancing the element of air until you become a flying dragoness.* All this energy enables you to take off. The dragoness lifts herself into the air. Let your shoulders and arms become wings, growing with every breath you take. Let your wing-arms swing higher and higher.

6. *Calmness and investigation of the prone, outstretched dragon-woman.* Calm down and stand still for a moment. Then lie down, get comfortable, and think about your movements and your voice. What did you learn about the dragon-woman within you? To which of her qualities would you like to give more space in your own life? Let yourself be a dreamer for a short while.

When you feel ready to return, take a couple more deep breaths, sprawl out, stretch, yawn—and when you open your eyes, you are a human woman again, one who carries all the experiences of the dragon-woman within her and can always relive them. With this in mind, get up and be on your way.

CREATIVE WAYS TO DEAL WITH STUMBLING BLOCKS
In the presence of one or more other people, it can easily happen that women want to "do it really well," so that a pressure to perform is added to the dancing elements; this tends to work against pleasurable, authentic self-expression. Sometimes it helps to consciously close your eyes and concentrate on your inner moods and impulses in order to create movements that correspond to your own feelings.

Another stumbling block can be making only "sparing" movements, so that no inner flame is fanned at all. In this case it can help to picture a wild, lustful, aggressive, and powerful dragoness, and to transform yourself into her by dancing. Remember, as with almost all movement meditations, the more energy you put in, the more experience you will gain.

🖎 Exercise 8: Saying good-bye to a young girl's self-limitation

Well before the emotional whirlwind of puberty, many young girls learn to limit themselves and their sexual feelings, adapting them to the ruling norms. The rest of the feelings are labeled unimportant: suppressed, denied, not even noticed. There are no words for their feelings, or else the words are devalued, twisted, or forbidden. In addition, for many, experiences of sexual violence, discrimination, or threats have linked feelings of fear, shame, guilt, and disgust to any kind of sexuality, and have made silence a quality necessary to survival. Therefore, girls often take on the "assignment" of repressing and limiting their desire, which affects them even as adult women.

GOAL
Identifying and limiting old (self-)repressive patterns.

STEP BY STEP
Make a written record here of your departure from self-limitation. Complete the following five sentences for yourself:

✳ I thought I couldn't ...

....

but now I learn that ...

....

✳ I always thought I was ...

....

but now I know that I ...

....

✳ I always thought I was supposed to ...

....

but now I know that it's much better for me if I ...

....

✳ My greatest fear was ...

....

but now I feel ...

....

✳ My conclusion for now and for later is ...

....

....

CREATIVE WAYS TO DEAL WITH STUMBLING BLOCKS

It is easy to make judgments and to evaluate people and to interpret things prematurely when dealing with others (especially if you don't know each other well enough yet). Instead, try out the magic word of love for once: "yes." Embrace a little "yes" for yourself, your history, your own way of being.

🐚 Exercise 9: Five questions about taking sexual responsibility

Many women try to pass the responsibility for their desires, their sexual satisfaction, and the activities that go along with them to someone else. However, sexual self-love is one of the places where I can learn the most about myself, and sexual encounters are where I can learn the most about my communication, my boundaries, and the combining of two love energies. This requires a knowledge of oneself and one's own body. In addition, my own dreams and fantasies contain important clues about my longings, needs, and borders. I could, of course, meditate on those things in my quiet little room, but sometimes it's easier and more productive to have an exchange with a receptive partner.

GOAL
An exchange with others about important questions of sexual self-love and sexual encounters in order to become more conscious of our own sexual identities as women.

TIME AND EXTERNAL PREPARATIONS
At least thirty minutes.

STEP BY STEP
Lie down comfortably, close together, so that you can whisper quietly to exchange your secrets. Use the following five questions as a prompt:

1. When do you remember experiencing your earliest encounter of sexual self-love? Explain using the present tense.

2. If you have orgasms, when and how was the first?

3. What are the important body parts that show you, from the outside, to be a sexual woman? What do you like about them and what do you dislike?

4. What are the taboos in your sexuality? What fantasies do you have that you don't (yet) dare to fulfill?

5. How would your life look in five years if, from now on, you were to make establishing an identity as a desiring, sexually satisfied

woman one of your most important goals and were to pursue it actively as well as passively?

CREATIVE WAYS TO DEAL WITH STUMBLING BLOCKS
If you come up against negative evaluations of yourself or the other person, it helps to concentrate on the questions and let the smart realist in you respond (instead of the norm-oriented judge). Furthermore, don't forget that your reality encompasses not only tangible facts, but also dreams, longings, and goals, as well as your talents and skills for reaching those goals. So take your dreams seriously, and use all your courage and creativity to take the next step in their direction!

VARIATIONS AND SUGGESTIONS
Shared in small groups, the answers to these five questions will not only create feelings of solidarity and connection, but can also free up even more creativity, particularly in terms of the steps needed to realize your dreams and visions of a life as a sexually fulfilled woman.

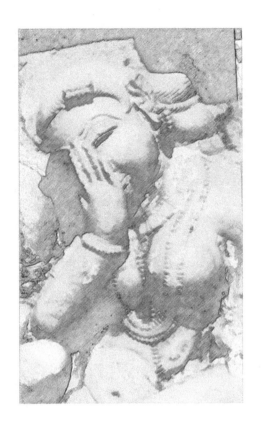

※ CHAPTER 4 ※

Fantasies in the Female Subconscious

*T*he activities and the meditation in this chapter encourage you to take responsibility for your own pleasure in a light and joyful way. You will automatically notice how fulfilling it can be to indulge yourself, your own imagination, and your knowing hands.

✎ Exercise 10: A creative trance-journey to your ideal inner beloved

The old saying "sex starts in the head" is still valid. If our skin, for example, is stroked with wonderful gentleness, we can only enjoy this sensation if we give the stroking the appropriate emotional coloring and meaning in our heads—if, that is, we have a loving, open relationship with the person whose hand is doing the stroking and if we find ourselves worthy of being stroked in this way. Then we not only open our pores and have our nerve endings ready to respond to even the most delicate stimuli, we can also couple the pleasant sensations with the appropriate feelings and pleasurable thoughts. Additionally, even just the idea of an inner beloved creates a certain inner satisfaction that makes us more independent from the neediness that "eats everything it can get." In short: The brain is another one of those body parts that makes better sex possible when it's well prepared and tuned in.

GOAL
Creating an inner picture of your ideal beloved and fusing spiritually with that being. This works against the female inclination toward modesty, which results in moderate sex, habitually the same. Instead, it promotes your concentration on dreams, visions, and innermost desires—which sometimes are not so unrealistic after all....

TIME AND EXTERNAL PREPARATIONS
About thirty minutes; find a thin mat that is not too soft; have a floor pillow and possibly a blindfold handy.

STEP BY STEP
* Stand on the mat and close your eyes (if necessary, use a blindfold).

✳ Lay a hand on your heart and use deep breaths to expand the space under your hand.

✳ Let all your thoughts, judgments, plans, etc., pass over you like white clouds. Or, if they are filling you up completely, stop providing them with energy, starting with your next breath. Instead, concentrate your energy on your feet. Feel how the soles of your feet are touching the floor. Start walking in place and making sounds (for example, sighing or growling, or a simple "aah" that flows out of your mouth as you exhale).

✳ Imagine that you are walking on a path. What does it look like? Is it rocky, level, or steep? Is it made of steaming asphalt, or is it a narrow path through the bushes? Look at it carefully! Smell the air and feel its warmth or its chill or the wind on your skin. What is to the right and left of the path? Houses? Landscapes? Look around, and walk, walk, walk.

✳ This is *your* path. Don't concentrate on an end point, just walk. Be aware of your entire body as you walk. Don't evaluate what you observe; simply observe even more closely what is moving and stirring within you.

✳ Walk in an upright posture and feel how your head becomes freer. Look into the distance and walk, one step at a time.

✳ Suddenly you see a figure appear! At first it's still tiny, shadowy, but it comes closer, step by step.

✳ You slowly approach one another. The other person becomes larger and more distinct. She or he appears to be very beautiful, something also emphasized through her or his clothing. As you get even closer to each other, you realize: This is the lover I've secretly always dreamed of! (Notice that the sex of the person created here by your imagination may or may not correspond to your sexual orientation. Open yourself to the possibility that even if you are heterosexual, your idealized lover in this fantasy can turn out to be female or vice versa.)

✳ Now that only a few yards separate you, you can see the other's perfect beauty, feel her or his captivating erotic aura, observe her or his supple movements. You smell the person's skin and feel the desire to love her or him on the spot, to melt into this person and become one.

✳ Do it—now! Stroke her, kiss her, undress her and yourself, allow yourself (and her) any movements, any sounds, and above all any feelings and sensations that you are capable of right now. Love him in every conceivable way, and give in completely to his caresses. This person knows you intimately, can sense what feels good to you right now, and does it before you even recognize the wish yourself. Your new lover is simply ideal! Play around, experiment, and try out everything that could be pleasurable for you, whether loud or quiet, tender or passionate, still or wild. (If you would rather sit or lie down for this part of the activity, do so.) Take the time to take in your new lover with all your senses, to melt together with this person.

✳ Then let yourselves grow calmer, and sit or lie next to one another for a moment, whatever feels right to you.

✳ Finally, say good-bye to your lover. And look: Your lover is giving you one last farewell gift as a memory of this wonderful encounter—one last embrace, a last kiss. Now you turn around at the same time as your lover and go back the way you came, step by step.

✳ While doing so, ask yourself: Which person out of my current environment or my past does this person resemble? Or is this person just the opposite—for example, the opposite of my current lover? Is she or he perhaps a secret part of myself?

✳ You should then ask yourself: How can I learn to accept the difference between this person and my real life? Has this encounter given me anything that could help me bring this person's kind of vitality into my real life? How do I feel after my encounter with my idealized lover?

✳ And while you are occupied with these questions, you come closer and closer to the starting point of your path. Having arrived, sit or lie down and allow yourself to review this experience for another moment.

✳ Now open your eyes. If you have been doing this exercise with a group, see if there's an individual near you with whom you would like to lie down and exchange your discoveries and experiences.

CREATIVE WAYS TO DEAL WITH STUMBLING BLOCKS

Many women shoot down their own imaginations by saying, "I couldn't follow through on that!" or, "Who would do that with me?" In these cases it sometimes helps to remember that the important thing is to discover and appreciate your own desires. After your trance-journey, as a second step, you can think about whether or not it is a fantasy you *want* to fulfill and, if so, how this could be achieved in the long term—in which relationship, with which resources, in what environment. Maybe you will determine that, practically speaking, you have to cross some things off your list, because some things simply aren't possible from an acrobatic standpoint. Still, you may find exciting new solutions if you put all your intelligence and creativity into fulfilling your wishes and dreams.

VARIATIONS AND SUGGESTIONS

If couples do this together, each can imagine that the ideal inner beloved is their partner. Then you can take this fantastic journey with the old and simultaneously newly discovered partner. When you report on it afterward to each other, it is important that the listening partner does not take the report as a set of instructions to be followed immediately; it should first be seen as the other person's dream or vision. Here, too, possible ways to implement the fantasy should only be considered as a second step.

🦢 Exercise 11: Erotic date

Who isn't familiar with this situation: feeling so sensual, beautiful, and seductive that this would be the perfect moment for an erotic encounter of the best kind. But where is your lover? That is still the great unknown. Squeezing yourself into that hot-looking, tight, sweaty leather outfit, you look through the events calendar to see if there's a singles' disco night somewhere (starting, of course, at a time of night when you, as a full-time worker bee, can only sip tiredly at a drink), or deciding whether you'll have to take in some cultural event in order to maybe chat up an interesting individual at the reception afterward just might be enough to transform your slight erotic vibration into nervous displeasure—and you turn on the TV. That works, too, but this is exactly the right time for the following game: Make a date! Make a date with a wonderful, tender, passionate woman who just happens to be in the mood: *Make a date with yourself!*

GOAL

In this game you can get to know yourself all over again and experience the autonomy of the self-loving woman who will do everything in her power to give you maximal sexual pleasure.

TIME AND EXTERNAL PREPARATIONS

At least thirty minutes, if possible open-ended. It is recommended that you prepare yourself and your love nest the way you would for the first night with a new lover (e.g., with candles, pillows, warmth, music, and pleasure-enhancing objects like feathers, flowers, etc.).

STEP BY STEP

* After you have set up the room nicely and maybe showered and put on some lotion, slowly undress and lie down comfortably on your bed.

* Lay one hand on your heart and the other on your belly or your pubic hair, and close your eyes.

* Imagine that, with the cunning anticipation, pubescent curiosity, and passionate desire of a red-blooded woman, you are meeting an exciting stranger who is just as aroused as you are.

* Since this person doesn't know you, you had better tell her or him everything you want them to know about you or be prepared for trial and error.

* Now switch back and forth between being the recipient and the giver of pleasure, and become more comfortable in each role. As

the recipient, give in totally; breathe the other person in deeply and allow yourself to make any sounds or movements that come to you. As pleasure-giver, stroke and caress your lover and enjoy every touch. You fulfill every desire that is acrobatically possible and allow yourself to enjoy the other's reactions.

* At the end, sink happily into one another until you become one person again and can enjoy the silence afterward without anyone wanting anything from you.

CREATIVE WAYS TO DEAL WITH STUMBLING BLOCKS

If you don't find yourself beautiful or erotic as a lover, imagine that this stranger finds you gorgeous and highly desirable. This person smiles at your attempts to contradict her or him. Do you jump nervously out of bed, or do you give it a try?

VARIATIONS AND SUGGESTIONS

This game can also be played wonderfully with two people, because you can make a mental date *with each other* (if possible, in different rooms at the same time) and pretend that you are together for the first time. I would postpone the discussion afterward until the next morning. It is important that the listener not associate what she hears with the stress of trying to do the exact same thing with her partner the next evening; the listener should understand the fantasy as her partner's "film." For the speaker, it is important that she give her partner so-called "undeserved compliments," such as, "Oh darling, last night you stroked my flanks so tenderly that little shouts of joy bubbled up out of me!" rather than nitpicking reproachfully. If you have an open and honest exchange, you give yourselves the chance, even after years together, to learn a lot about the other person and your own reactions.

🍃 Exercise 12: Fantastical self-arousal

This exercise goes a step further than the creative trance-journey, in that the fantasies and dreams don't remain in your head, but rather spread out into your whole body—without the help of any kind of "handiwork" (like the kind used on the "Erotic date").

GOAL

Physical self-arousal without any kind of touching—just with your imagination and your breathing.

TIME AND EXTERNAL PREPARATIONS

About thirty minutes; a soft mat and a blanket.

STEP BY STEP

* Lie down or sit comfortably; cover yourself if you like. Close your eyes and concentrate on your breathing: Breathe in deeply—and out again—with the knowledge that with each breath you are drawing new vitality into yourself. When breathing out, let yourself go; let go of your tension, and let yourself come into your own rhythm until it's easy to let your inhalation and exhalation come and go like waves on the ocean. This is the breath of pleasure, the breath of simple ecstasy.

* As you continue to breathe in this way, go for a stroll in your inner self—enter the world of erotic images and fantasies. Do you feel what it's like in this place? What do you see? What do you hear? How is the light here? Is the room big and open or small and intimate? Whatever may wait for you here, just let it come toward you. And if something bothers you, just forcefully push out the disturbance as you exhale.

* As you are breathing calmly, go into this room of sensual pictures and become acquainted with it. And when you are ready, approach the pictures and imaginings that give you an erotic tingle, that arouse you. Look around until you find some. Instead of pictures, it might be sounds or movements or a feeling, a specific memory, or a physical sensation. Whatever it is, breathe it in completely. Deeply. And breathe it out. And in again. As though this imagining could glide through you.

* Now begin to react to the images and feelings that arouse you. Let yourself be aroused, breathe into them, let yourself go—give in completely to the pleasurable thought. And remember, this place inside you belongs to you alone! Everything is in your hands here.

In this place, open up to yourself and feel completely conscious. Give in to the arousal that you feel in every cell of your body. Give in to the arousal as you dive into your fantasies—as you breathe in and out more and more deeply. Allow yourself to feel what happens in your body, your soul, your spirit, in every part of you when you accept your inner arousal. Allow yourself to increase your arousal with every breath, to let it spread out inside you. Allow yourself to acknowledge and enjoy being aroused. Maybe you feel like an open, flesh-eating plant. Maybe you are the ocean that comes and goes in waves. Maybe you are the sun, opening your arms and embracing the green earth. Whatever and however you might be right now, breathe in and out deeply.

✳ Allow yourself to linger in this place of arousal, of pleasurable pictures and sensations.

✳ Then give it one last glance and get ready to return to the present, to the outside world. Let your breathing grow calmer again and say good-bye to this place. After all, you know you can come back here any time.

✳ Finally, move around and stretch before you open your eyes and get up.

CREATIVE WAYS TO DEAL WITH STUMBLING BLOCKS
Even in the fantasy world, the old norms and values can sometimes intrude. Therefore, you may prevent yourself from becoming aroused by reactivating old taboos or by expecting yourself to become aroused immediately. It usually helps to take a deep breath and imagine that you are forcefully breathing out all of your old expectations, taboos, commandments, judgments, and thoughts about "right" and "wrong." Allow yourself to recognize yourself a little more clearly with each breath and to accept your sensations and feelings the way they are right now.

It may also be that you drift off into destructive, torturous victim fantasies, or that you suffer from the thought of all the pleasurable sex you've missed out on in the past. If so, remember that your body is more "generous" than your mind, and maybe it doesn't feel like sitting in the corner and moping anymore. Maybe a little arousal without too much contact and touching is exactly what your wounded and not-yet-healed heart needs.

VARIATIONS AND SUGGESTIONS

If it's possible for you to do this exercise in an open and protected spot in nature, you may feel more closely connected to nature's pulse. This exercise can also become more intense with each repetition.

✒ Exercise 13: Through the ocean's depths with the dolphin-woman

Dolphins are very intelligent and sensitive animals that are full of vitality, a sense of community, playfulness, joy, and trust.

GOAL

Strengthening the water element, or the feeling element, within you. This happens when you trustingly let yourself be led into supportive fantasy worlds and accept yourself however you might be feeling just then. The more well-intentioned you are, and the more you seriously allow yourself to be as you really are, the deeper and more intense this encounter with yourself will be.

TIME AND EXTERNAL PREPARATIONS

At least an hour. If you record the following step-by-step text onto a tape first, it may be easier for you to relax while listening.

STEP BY STEP

* Sit down comfortably and close your eyes. Make sure that your spine is straight and your hands are lying loosely on the tops of your thighs; your thumbs and index fingers are gently and lightly touching.

* Now take a few deep breaths in and out, and with every exhalation feel how everything that is heavy or dark is falling away from you. As you breathe, feel how your breathing begins to flow more easily and lightly. Observe your breath; pay attention as you breathe in and out. Your breath rises within you like a silver column and

leaves you like the whisper of a summer wind. With every breath out, feel how you are sinking deeper and deeper into relaxed calmness.

✳ As you continue to breathe regularly, observe your body. Is there tension in any of your muscles? If you feel any, breathe in; when you breathe out, release the tension. Let your breath flow through the tense muscles and become softer.

✳ Now shift your attention to your labia, and imagine that roots are growing out of them. They grow deep and broad, and they penetrate more and more deeply through all the earth's layers. With your imagination, follow these roots until you reach their end. Here a deep cave is opened up for you. It is light enough that you are able to look around. As you let your eyes wander around the cave, you see some drinking vessels on the left side. On the vessels is the inscription "liquid light." Allow yourself to taste it, and then drink pure liquid light out of one of these vessels. Feel how the light flows into you, through all of your muscles and nerves. The light flows through every cell of your body. Feel how brightness and lightness flow through you. How does this feel?

✳ Everything around you grows brighter, and you notice an exit. You walk out of the cave and come upon a long beach. A boundless sky stretches out over your head. Can you feel the fresh ocean air and the vastness in and above you? Let yourself breathe freely and deeply.

✳ The ocean's waves come and go—and you watch how the water flows up and then ebbs again. After a while you decide to walk carefully into the water. Is it warm enough? Slowly, step by step, you go in, and as it gets deeper, you begin to swim effortlessly. Relax as you swim in the vastness of the ocean.

✳ Suddenly a dolphin surfaces next to you. She greets you and invites you to climb onto her back. You do so and put your arms around her in order to hold on. Now you are swimming together in the far reaches of the ocean.

* After a while, she takes you down into the depths of the ocean.
  You're amazed that you can breathe under water as well. Can you
  trust yourself and the dolphin? Can you give yourself over to her
  guidance? Dare to do it! Let yourself be carried by the dolphin-
  woman. You swim together past colorful schools of fish and
  through glowing coral reefs. Your eyes adjust to the light in this
  mysterious and diverse underwater world.

* Suddenly, in the distance, you see a silvery shimmer of light. It is
  made up of dancing points of light that grow larger and larger,
  and you realize it is a group of many dolphins. They swim toward
  you, play with you, accompany you. It's as though pure joy were
  emanating from them. They play with you as though that were the
  whole point of their existence, to enjoy themselves with you. And
  you hear a soft whisper: "We're going to swim to the heart of the
  earth, where only love lives."

* Maybe you can't imagine that yet; maybe you feel a longing or
  curiosity within you. And as you keep swimming, you see a glowing pyramid in the middle of the ocean, with an entrance that
  glows even more brightly. You swim around it a few times. Then
  you gently glide off your dolphin's back and go though the
  entrance into the pyramid. Observe the energy, the light, the
  atmosphere inside. Look, smell, listen, feel.

* Then a gentle voice reaches your ear like soft waves: "I welcome
  you to the central chamber of the earth's heart—here, where only
  love lives."

* Your eyes slowly adjust to the brightness, and you see a glowing
  figure offering you a glass filled with the essence of love. The
  figure speaks to you: "You have come here to experience the wavelength of joy and love. This elixir has been prepared for you in
  order to heighten your vibrations, take away your fatigue, and
  dissolve your sorrows. Take this glass and drink." You take the glass
  and drink the pleasant-tasting elixir. You feel love rising up within
  you and harmony enveloping you.

✳ Take a minute to let this state of love and joy spread through you, and to enjoy the silence of the moment. Then thank the figure for the wondrous elixir and take your leave. You know that you can come back to this place of love and joy anytime.

✳ You leave the pyramid, and your dolphin-woman is happily waiting for you outside. You climb onto her back again, and again you swim together through the vastness of the ocean—past glowing coral reefs and colorful schools of fish—until finally you return to the water's surface.

✳ Now you say good-bye to your dolphin, and you swim the rest of the way back to the beach alone. You walk along the beach to your cave's entrance. In the cave, you lay a hand on your heart and feel how the essence of love is spreading from your heart through your whole body, shining out into the cave and raining back down onto you as little sparks of joy.

✳ Then decide whether you want to leave your heart open or close it up a little for your journey back to the top. Return upward along the roots that reach into the cave. Once you have arrived, you can pull your roots back up and let them disappear into your labia.

✳ Now comes the most important step, the one that turns the fantasy journey into a meditation: Linger in peace for a little while and find the stillness within you.

✳ Breathe in and out deeply a few times, and let yourself return gradually to waking consciousness.

✳ Move your limbs: first your feet, then your hands, then your arms and legs. Open your eyes and stretch. Feel how you gradually arrive completely in the here and now.

CREATIVE WAYS TO DEAL WITH STUMBLING BLOCKS

It may be that a woman drifts into distressing, negative fantasies. If so, maybe only consciously halting her train of thought will help—breathing deeply and powerfully, and consciously creating new images. After the meditation, it may be worthwhile to think about what it means that these distressing images came up for you. But doing this *during* the meditation negates the intended effect.

For some, this fantasy journey may contain too many images. Shorten the trip however you like, and follow only the suggestions that fit into the flow of your own current fantasy world.

VARIATIONS AND SUGGESTIONS

The phase of playing together in the ocean can be lengthened, especially if you have had real encounters with dolphins and want to luxuriate in those memories a little longer.

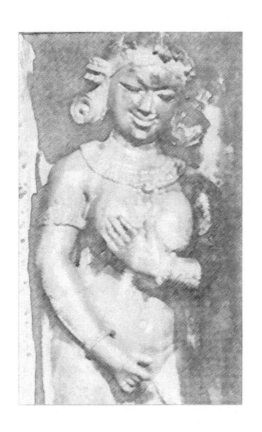

Wild and Tender
Games with Yourself

*T*he suggestions that follow for playing with yourself will give you even more concrete incentives to enlarge and broaden your sexual potential. As already described in the deep-breathing portion of the tuning-in session (see "Six Keys to the Gates of Physical Pleasure" in Chapter 3, page 55), your breath here will play the role of a flying carpet that can carry you up high into the sky and gently let you touch down again. Exercise 17, "Gladdening the heart," is adapted from the sky-dancing tantrikas of the Cherokee Indian tradition. It offers insights (that can be experienced with the body) into the manifold possibilities of spreading and transforming sexual energy. (For more about this, see also Chapters 7 and 10.)

🦋 Exercise 14: The art of panting

As you have seen in many of these exercises, breathing is the thread on which all of these colorful love beads are strung. The deeper and longer your breaths are, the stronger the thread grows. When you take breaths that are about three times as deep as usual, you take in more oxygen than you need. This builds up your energy field, an electromagnetically charged field that gives you protection and strength.

This way of breathing may be familiar to you from intense, arousing sexual encounters. By concentrating on it consciously here, you can increase your sensations and enjoy them more intensely. Sexual panting is not just a powerful cleansing technique for all your breathing organs, but also serves to spread sexual energy throughout your body and your surroundings.

GOAL

Practicing deep, powerful, conscious chest and stomach breathing, thereby working on the basic activity that creates both the physical requirements for pleasurable sexuality and the mental requirements for actively recognizing what exists. Concretely, this means opening the channel between your vulva/labia and your mouth/upper lips. You will learn that you can "breathe through your vulva" just as well as through your mouth. It is a way to connect consciousness with vertical breathing. The exercise strengthens your sensual and erotic perceptions (tasting, feeling, etc.) and helps spread them through your entire body.

TIME AND EXTERNAL PREPARATIONS
About twenty minutes.

STEP BY STEP

* ✳ Sit down comfortably, close your eyes, and lay one hand like a bowl over your vulva/yoni. Lay your other hand on top of it.

* ✳ Then breathe in, moving your second hand from your yoni to your mouth.

* ✳ Now breathe out, and let your hand glide back down from your mouth to your yoni.

* ✳ As you are tracing the channel between your upper lips and lower labia with your hand, along the front of your body, imagine the channel inside you. Imagine it opening up. These kinds of "imaginings" can help you actually "form an image" inside your body, causing a real physical change (as has been proven, for example, in research on autogenic practice).

* ✳ Begin with sexual breathing, otherwise known as *wind-sucking*. Breathe as if you were breathing in through a big straw, with a soft sucking noise. Breathe in with your mouth loosely open, and breathe out with a stretched-out "aaahh."

* ✳ First, concentrate on the two lip levels (the mouth's lips and the labia), one after the other. Then concentrate more on your labia and imagine their inhalations and exhalations.

* ✳ After fifteen or twenty minutes, yawn, stretch, and open your eyes again.

CREATIVE WAYS TO DEAL WITH STUMBLING BLOCKS
Shallow breathing: Here it may help to see what happens if you imagine simply inhaling three times as much air as usual.

Another stumbling block can be *forced breathing (hyperventilation),* and the dizziness that can result. For this, it helps to emphasize a longer exhalation as well as overall relaxation and attempting to use your hands or whole body to make more contact with the earth. For advanced cases of hyperventilation, it helps to breathe in your own exhalation (by cupping your hands in front of your face), to grip other hands or objects, or to have your back stroked by a helpful person who can also demonstrate slow breathing.

It may be that at first you don't have a clear feeling for the different breathing levels. It doesn't matter—sexual breathing doesn't care how much your brain understands. Be patient.

VARIATIONS AND SUGGESTIONS
You can expand this exercise by beginning to open the channel between your yoni and your crown chakra. This happens as if by accident when you send your inhalation to the top of your head first—pause in your breathing—wait until the exhalation comes by itself and send it deep into the ground—take another break in your breathing—wait until the inhalation comes by itself and send it back up to the top of your head (or even six inches or so higher). This is a way to lengthen your consciousness beyond the vertical boundaries of your body, so that you can experience stretching between heaven and earth more and more clearly, and you can feel your greatness as a woman.

Exercise 15: Sexual breathing

This breathing exercise is a deepening of the previous one. The effect—in combination with self-love or love-play with a partner—can be very ecstatic and border-dissolving. But even without this connection, the exercise promotes a clear sense that you stretch between heaven and earth.

Another effect of this exercise is that your sensual and erotic perceptions (taste, feeling, etc.) are strengthened and spread more throughout your whole body. If you practice sexual breathing in your lovemaking, a new world of broadened pleasure will open up for you.

GOAL
Playing even more easily with moving your breath vertically, in a fiery way.

TIME AND EXTERNAL PREPARATIONS
Anywhere between fifteen minutes and the long period of time spent in love games, where you can repeatedly remind yourself to concentrate on this kind of breathing. Use a soft mat.

STEP BY STEP

* ✳ Lie down comfortably and take a few deep breaths, emphasizing the exhalation.

* ✳ Then relax your neck and head a little by massaging them yourself, and lift and swivel your head very gently (five minutes).

* ✳ Next, your pelvic floor is dynamically loaded while you remain lying on your back, but now with your knees bent. Your feet should remain completely on the floor. Then lift your pelvis and "pound" it gently (!) on the floor, making sounds as you do so (five to ten minutes).

* ✳ Then begin your sexual breathing, sucking in air as if through a wide straw and breathing it out through your opened mouth. Bend your knees a little more. Then, *while breathing in,* draw energy in through your labia. Purse your mouth's lips a little to make a sound like the wind, and tip your pelvic floor back a little in order to create a slight arch in your lower back. Your hands accompany your breathing motion by gliding from your root chakra through your whole body to your crown chakra. It's as though you were pulling energy and air upward with your hands and through the contractions of your genital muscles. *While breathing out,* let your hands wander from your crown chakra back to your yoni as you let the crown chakra's energy flow through the root chakra, pushing it out with your genital muscles. While doing this, tip your pelvis forward, rounding your back a little (fifteen to twenty minutes).

CREATIVE WAYS TO DEAL WITH STUMBLING BLOCKS

If you are with a partner, she may be alienated by your breathing technique. It's best to explain ahead of time what you intend to do.

When you're alone, allow yourself to experiment and play around a little without using the sexual breathing perfectly all the time.

VARIATIONS AND SUGGESTIONS

If you want, you can also go into an exercise with your partner called the "jellyfish": Your partner sits behind you the whole time with your head between her legs and holds your hands. You look into each other's eyes, and you give in to your body's spontaneous feelings and movements (fifteen to twenty minutes or more).

The next time, you can also try the "butterfly": While breathing in, open your knees, which are still bent, and close them as you breathe out. Your legs and your yoni open and close like the wings of a butterfly.

⚗ *Exercise 16: Opening the inner flute*

The inner flute is an image developed by Margot Anand for the human being's chakra system (see Chapter 2). The image implies that your own breath and your energy space are like the reed or bamboo flute, whose notes are produced by playing on its holes/funnels (analogous to the chakras) and create the individuality of each person. The inner flute is a magical instrument through which all the chakras can be connected by the air you breathe. If you channel sexual energy through the flute from the depths of your lap, you spread the fire of love through your whole body. Since most human flutes are blocked in various places by painful, frightening, or restrictive experiences, there are many exercises to free up the flow of breathing and life energy. (Two examples are "Fire-breathing orgasm," Exercise 46, and "The chakra wave," Exercise 31.) These exercises work best when we use the first key to the gates of physical pleasure (maximally deepened breathing) and the third key (allowing various sounds and noises that can help rid the body of spiritual, mental, and physical waste matter). (See "Six Keys to the Gates of Physical Pleasure," in Chapter 3, page 55.)

GOAL

Becoming conscious of the inner channel through the middle of your body, along your spine between the pelvic floor and the brain. We open this channel, the inner flute, by combining the following elements:

* deep breathing through the open mouth,

* pelvic movements,

* visualization (i.e., picturing something as an image).

When the flute is open, energy moves through the body and connects the chakras, and then we are able to feel and enjoy great pleasure and energy. This breathing opens the door for orgasms that take hold of the entire body, as well as orgasms that extend beyond the body.

TIME AND EXTERNAL PREPARATIONS

Ten to twenty minutes. You can stand up or lie down while doing the exercise. If you want to lie down, you will need a mat or mattress.

STEP BY STEP

* ✳ First, create an inner picture of the chakras as funnel-shaped energy wheels in your aura—especially along the front of your body. Then breathe through your opened mouth and imagine that you are breathing deeply through your pelvis or through your labia.

* ✳ Once you have the feeling that your whole pelvic and yoni area is awakened, well circulated, and flexible, you can begin to make small movements of the pelvis (e.g., a tiny tilting motion or a delicate vibration) and consciously increase them.

* ✳ Now go through the chakras one by one, and for each one imagine that you are breathing mostly through this lower flute hole. As you breathe in, take in fresh air; and as you breathe out, get rid of any tensions or other unpleasant feelings, and accompany their release with screeching, moaning, or any other sounds that you find helpful. When you reach the crown chakra, imagine a large channel running between your crown and your labia (or your perineum), and take a few deep breaths from top to bottom and from bottom to top.

* ✳ Next, let your breathing grow calmer and quieter. While doing so, you might imagine that you are breathing in deeply through your labia and pulling the breath up to your crown. Hold an inhalation for a few moments. When you feel the impulse to exhale, breathe all the way back down and out through your labia, and pause for another few seconds until the impulse to breathe in causes you to pull your breath upward again.

* Once this way of breathing has become easier for you, you can concentrate especially on the pauses at the top and bottom, and feel what is happening to you.

CREATIVE WAYS TO DEAL WITH STUMBLING BLOCKS
It may be that in these breathing pauses you feel beset by a strange uneasiness, or possibly you drift off into stressful thoughts. If so, concentrate your entire awareness on what is happening to your body during these breaks from breathing.

VARIATIONS AND SUGGESTIONS
For some women it may be useful to do a grounding exercise after this breathing exercise, in order to keep from "losing yourself." For example, lie flat on your stomach and lay your palms on the floor, concentrating on your contact with the earth; or do the exercise "In the lap of Mother Earth," Exercise 2.

Exercise 17: Gladdening the heart

This exercise, developed by the Cherokee women, is an excellent way to draw power from self-love and distribute it through the entire body. The basis of the exercise is a teaching about sexual-spiritual life energy called Quodoushka. This age-old knowledge has only been passed on to us in recent years because of the threat of the Cherokee tribe's extinction.

The term *Quodoushka* refers to the spiritual energy that is created when two Chuluaques, life-force energies, come together and create a new quality of energy. The openness of this teaching is demonstrated by the fact that these two life-force energies do not, out of "physical necessity," need to belong to different genders. On the contrary, the Cherokee women proceed from the assumption that the feminine always includes the masculine, not the other way around. However, this connection to the power of female existence has become more and more torn by the rise of male power through patriarchy, and even women themselves are no longer able to recognize and honor their own sexual magnetism and that of "Grandmother Earth." In order to divert further harm from themselves and from nature, the Cherokee women teach us how to step out of the role of victim, encounter our inner child with healing, reactivate our sexual power, and let sexual magnetism work for us and for the advancement of all living things.

GOAL

Overcoming old patterns of dependency in sex and energetically charging your whole body.

TIME AND EXTERNAL PREPARATIONS

It's a good idea to plan at least an hour for the actual game with yourself and to arrange beforehand a sensual, familiar, and beautiful love nest in a warm room free of telephones or other distractions.

STEP BY STEP

* This game with yourself starts out with good old "freestyle." This means you should stroke and pamper yourself in all the places that especially take in and distribute your erotic energy. (See also "Self-love ritual in the presence of another," Exercise 43, or parts of "MMM: Magic 'mussel' massage," Exercise 48.) Play with yourself, tease, tempt, and arouse yourself, and play with your clitoris to bring yourself to the edge of ecstasy. (This doesn't necessarily have to be the "classic" orgasm; it could simply be a nice, high level of arousal.)

* For those who lean toward orgasmic forms of ecstasy: Just before the "point of no return," that is, before you let yourself fall into an orgasm, take a deep breath and guide your sexual fire out of your pearl, out of your lap, into your heart level. Feel for a moment as though your heart is filled with fire from the level of your pelvis—and just as you begin to feel comfortably relaxed, start to arouse yourself all over again, and fan your fire anew.

* For those who don't experience orgasms in the classic sense: Simply place yourself in a state of high arousal; bring this arousal to the heart level with a deep breath; become aware of it; and just before you become comfortably relaxed, begin the self-arousal again.

* The Cherokee women suggest doing this four times in a row.
  Then, the fifth time, let yourself fall into your orgasm or your
  particular form of ecstasy.

CREATIVE WAYS TO DEAL WITH STUMBLING BLOCKS

For women who don't usually have multiple orgasms, this exercise can create similar performance pressure. You can reduce it by resolving to *play*
with the exercise rather than stimulating yourself in order to reach a clear
orgasmic experience.

VARIATIONS AND SUGGESTIONS

In order to use the healing power of this energy combination (of arousal
and relaxation), you might draw your sexual fire upward with a deep breath
(not just to the heart level, but into sick or injured body parts) and leave it
there as you breathe out. This is only recommended if you need more energy in those body parts to improve their circulation, vitality, and strength.
If certain body parts already have too much energy, it may be more helpful to steer your sexual fire toward a part of the body that is farthest away,
to balance the flow of energy.

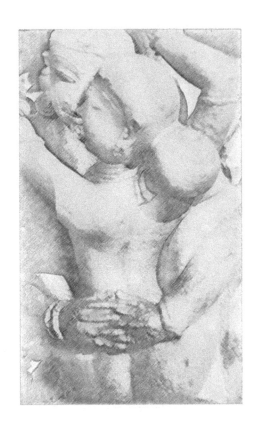

⇜ CHAPTER 6 ⇝

Games and Exercises
for Two

*B*y now you are fairly advanced in the pleasurable forms of sexual self-responsibility. But how does it work with another person—someone whom you may love or like but who is so darned different, with different wishes, needs, rhythms, and energy flows? Well, tantra offers wondrous recipes that can succeed with a tablespoon of patience, a teaspoon of humor, and some of the following exercises. With their help, the differences between you and your beloved can be accepted, and with a wink and with loving thoughtfulness, both partners' energy states can come together in one shared vibration.

✌ Exercise 18: Pulling stress out of her

As I have already mentioned, stressed-out women's souls usually need relief, then relaxation, and finally enough impulses to build up any erotic energy at all. In this consumption-oriented age, fewer and fewer people want to do this "regenerative work" themselves; instead, they want someone to do it for them. This exercise teaches you to pull out each other's stress.

GOAL
Using this simple stretching and shaking massage exercise, stress-related knots in your muscles and joints are loosened a little, making the path clearer for your subtle erotic-sexual energy.

TIME AND EXTERNAL PREPARATIONS
About forty-five minutes for each partner; however, shorter versions are also possible (it's better to leave out individual parts than not to relax at all). Have a blanket handy, if desired.

STEP BY STEP
  * After you have agreed on who will receive the massage first, the pleasure recipient lies down on a firm mat or carpeted floor and breathes out deeply and audibly with an "aahh."

  * *Instructions for the active partner, or "pleasure guide":* Begin with a gentle touch on the enjoyer's belly and one on the heart chakra, and adjust your breathing to that of the enjoyer.

✳ Now squat comfortably near your partner's head, cross your hands, and lay each hand on one of your partner's shoulders. As you exhale, lean on your partner's shoulders with about half of your weight (if you're very light, use even more of your weight), pushing the shoulders down and outward a little bit. The pleasure recipient breathes out slowly with an "aahh."

✳ Now reach under your partner's shoulder blades (work your way under them until your hands lie beneath the "wings"), and begin to shake them from underneath as hard as you can. The pleasure recipient allows this, but can of course say "Stop" at any time if she doesn't like something.

✳ Now sit next to your partner's right side, and gradually begin to stretch and to shake her right arm, from her hand to her lower arm to her shoulder joint. Repeat this step with the left arm.

✳ Place yourself at your partner's waist, take both of her hands, and shake her arms simultaneously, varying the strength and speed of the shaking. This calls for the wild, playful child in you! If the pleasure recipient doesn't like something, she will tell you. Meanwhile, bring a little chaos into her body! The recipient will thank you. After you've shaken out her arms, lay them carefully down and stroke them, one after the other, from top to bottom.

✳ Now do the same thing with your partner's legs. To shake them, you need to find a good stance so you can use your full strength. Before you lay down the legs, pull them forcefully, stretching them out. After laying them down, firmly hold the soles of the feet to give your partner a sense of peace and security.

✳ Now sit at your partner's head. Hold her neck with one hand and her forehead with the other for a little while, using a firmness that the recipient should determine.

✳ Next, if she likes, cover your partner with a blanket and leave her alone for a few minutes while she investigates the chaos of the various effects this exercise has had on her body.

CREATIVE WAYS TO DEAL WITH STUMBLING BLOCKS

Pleasure guides are often uncertain about what force and speed are appropriate when shaking the pleasure recipient's limbs. Don't worry—it's the recipient's job to tell you if she doesn't like something, and how she would rather have you do it. What if some recipients don't want to criticize and therefore don't say anything? Too bad. Does that mean she missed her chance to feel the right touch? No, because there's always a next time....

VARIATIONS AND SUGGESTIONS

Once your recipient is nicely open and relaxed, it means her tension has been removed. As her pleasure guide, give her something else in exchange. For example, gentle stroking, a warm breath on bare skin, teasing sensitive areas with ostrich feathers (you can get cheap ones in craft stores), or whatever else occurs to your playful self and doesn't meet with any resistance.

🌿 Exercise 19: Letting yourself be comfortably flattened

This exercise prepares the massaging partner to give a relaxation massage that involves working not with force, but with one's weight. It prepares the person being massaged to rely on her own connection to the earth as well as on the other person's weight.

GOAL

Relaxation for both receiver and giver.

TIME AND EXTERNAL PREPARATIONS

About ten to twenty minutes. A medium-soft mat is best.

STEP BY STEP

* *If you're the pleasure recipient,* lie down on your stomach and breathe in and out deeply a few times. Emphasize the outward breath and imagine that with each exhalation you are sinking deeper and deeper into the mat, growing flatter and flatter.

* *If you are the massaging partner, or giver,* sit by the recipient's side for a moment and breathe along with her. While doing so, relax and imagine that both you and your partner will soon sink farther into the earth.

✳ Begin to lower the weight of your upper body onto the recipient's buttocks, leaning on your hands and outstretched arms. Pause for a few seconds, and then release your hands in order to move down the recipient's legs, using the same grip. The recipient can use sounds or even words to communicate which pressure points feel good and where the pressure is too strong or too weak. In any case, any sounds made during this process are relaxing. As you continue to press your partner's legs into the ground, be careful to use only your weight, not your strength. It's also important that you use only a very small amount of pressure on the recipient's joints (knees, ankles, etc.) and that you are also gentle with the tendons attached to them. The larger the muscle group, the more weight you can place on it.

✳ When you reach the recipient's soles, you can get up and stand close to the feet; your own heels rest on the ground while the front part of your soles rest on the recipient's soles. Here, too, it is important to discuss how much weight feels pleasantly relaxing.

✳ Next, squat down and begin to place weight on the recipient's legs, but this time with your hands or legs, sitting down or even rolling over the recipient with your whole body, stopping just below the neck. The kidney region should be treated with caution; other than that, the lower and middle back can usually bear a lot of weight as long as it is spread out evenly across the muscle tissue. This can develop into a game where you try to use your weight and as many body parts as possible to help the recipient sink into the ground.

✳ Afterward, if the recipient likes, she can turn over and have the entire process—very carefully—repeated on her front side. It is important that weight be placed on the recipient's belly very slowly at first, and that weight on the rib cage be spread out, possibly by you sitting on it. Be sure to press the recipient's shoulders into the ground with your hands and upper body weight.

✳ It is easier for you to administer your weight as you exhale; it's also nice for the recipient if her breathing is synchronized with your breath, so that she can breathe into the stretch.

CREATIVE WAYS TO DEAL WITH STUMBLING BLOCKS

Some givers are too cautious and lessen the relaxing effect by applying too little weight; some are so excited by all the possibilities presented by muscle groups and fat pillows that they may fail to sense what feels good to the recipient. In both cases, the most important thing is to communicate with each other, using words if necessary, in order to prevent misunderstandings.

VARIATIONS AND SUGGESTIONS

This exercise can also be done by three people, which gives the recipient an exciting sense of confusion. In the end, she will hardly know who is pressing on her where and how, and, if the two givers are well coordinated, the recipient will be able to relax her body even farther into the ground. This variation does take longer, but it usually increases the pleasure of all three participants.

◌ Exercise 20: Letting go of feelings

If we want to postpone pleasurable and ecstatic sexuality until we've worked through all of our potentially troubling feelings, either through psychotherapy or some other way, we may grow older and wiser, but we'll miss out on all the pleasure that's possible without undergoing these processes. Here's a little exercise that helps transform destructive feelings and inclines us toward contact within the moment.

GOAL

Letting go of old emotional ties in order to be free for feelings of love in the moment.

TIME AND EXTERNAL PREPARATIONS

About twenty minutes for each partner.

STEP BY STEP

* *Enjoyer,* lie down on your back and breathe out with an audible sigh.

* *Giver,* first touch the recipient's heart on the right side and ask what she feels there. *Enjoyer,* investigate and make room for all the

feelings that surface, letting them come more and more strongly into your consciousness. Then release the feelings by breathing out, giving them a sound and setting them free in space, or by expressing them through a motion and allowing your spirit to set them free.

* Now, *giver*, do the same with the left side of the recipient's heart, the solar plexus, the navel, and the root chakra.

* Afterward, the recipient can take a moment to meditate in silence; the giver no longer touches her but remains inwardly bound to her.

* Now switch roles. Only after the exercise is over do you have a brief exchange with each other about the experience.

CREATIVE WAYS TO DEAL WITH STUMBLING BLOCKS
Very shallow breathing can cause a shallower recognition of all our feelings. Sometimes it helps to have the giver breathe audibly along with the recipient in order to encourage deeper breathing. Nevertheless, the recipient's breathing should not be forced by the application of physical pressure on the spots mentioned above.

Another stumbling block can result if you work yourself up into a particular feeling; in this case, the giver no longer has the impression that the recipient has the feeling; instead, it seems like the *feeling has taken hold of the recipient*. If so, it's a good idea to gently point out to her that she can let go of this feeling for the moment, even if she will deal with it again later and try to understand it better or express it more thoroughly.

VARIATIONS AND SUGGESTIONS
Sometimes mixed emotions—or, rather than clear emotions, pictures, colors, or sounds—will come up. It can be helpful to describe these pictures, to feel out and investigate their contents, in order to let go of them again as you breathe out.

🐚 Exercise 21: Lioness, sow, mosquito

In contrast to many women's fears that aggressive energy is always destructive, this exercise shows that anger or frustration, for example, are really just expansive, fiery types of energy. If you have internal and external permission to feel this kind of firepower, and to express it without hurting yourself or others, it can be experienced as pleasurable (rather than threatening). Besides, physically expressing aggression increases vitality and raises your overall energy level (by aiding the flow of energy and freeing up energy that is usually used for repressing things). This creates more room for sexual energy as well. In addition, the red, wild power of the woman is made up of sex *and* aggression! We cannot make a clean distinction between them. However, we can steer their expression into particular paths and cultivate their power. We begin by coaxing these energy forces out and, like children imitating animals, playing with them rather than immediately asking ourselves to express them in an "adult," coherent, and effective way.

GOAL

Playing with the lustful-aggressive side of our energy by expressing it in animal roles.

TIME AND EXTERNAL PREPARATIONS

About thirty minutes for all three kinds of animals combined. A firm mat, on which both people can squat and move around, is a good idea. A glass of water can be placed at a safe distance to quench your thirst after the lioness phase. For amateur screamers, it's nice to have a cough drop for the relaxation phase.

STEP BY STEP

* *Lioness:* The theme embodied by the lioness is "Get the aggression out!" Each partner takes on the qualities they imagine to be part of a strong, wild, battle-ready lioness. You can make threatening gestures and approach the other aggressively; you can growl, squint, stick out your tongue, put out your claws, lunge forward as you breathe out, and express all the aggression you have available, all without touching the other person or hurting her with words.

* *Sow:* The theme of the sow is "Eat everything up!" Each partner imagines that they are a hungry sow, looking for truffles and other delicacies, wallowing in the dirt, and finding something to eat there. Pull up your shoulders, turn everything inward instead of

out, breathe noisily through your nose, and draw your breath upward. Then sniff every bend and fold of the other person, "looking for truffles" in every hidden little corner of their body. Curious touches with your nose are allowed, but confining contact with the arms or legs is not.

* *Mosquito:* The theme of the mosquito is "Draw all sounds and energies into your own center and let yourself be carried by their flight." Here, each of you imagines that you are a mosquito (maybe even a hungry one) who can only fly with the help of the sounds you make. Breathe in deeply and imagine that the sound is especially concentrated in the upper part of your head. Then breathe out with a very high-pitched noise. While doing this you can get on the other person's nerves by buzzing around their head like a bloodthirsty mosquito. The other person, of course, does the same, so both are in motion at the same time.

* Afterward, sit down facing each other and close your eyes for a moment in order to let the three kinds of aggression you've experienced sink in. Then spend a little time comparing your experiences.

CREATIVE WAYS TO DEAL WITH STUMBLING BLOCKS
Some people try to trivialize real feelings of aggression as they come up by laughing or "being nice." Again, the same rule holds true here: Give in totally so you will be able to come away with an authentic experience.

People may also be easily frightened by anothers' aggression, and freeze. It is important to encourage yourself—or let yourself be encouraged—to actively defend yourself and to attack as well (especially in the role of the lioness).

VARIATIONS AND SUGGESTIONS
As always, it's important to make sure there are no physical injuries (especially in the lioness phase) while at the same time activating your own creativity enough to make maximal aggressive expression possible.

One possible variation is to do the same exercise with several people in a circle. You all embody the lioness at the same time, then the sow, and finally the mosquito. This is less frightening for some women, but possibly less effective than a direct confrontation with one person.

〰 Exercise 22: Dance of the she-demons

Who isn't familiar with this situation? You're hot for each other, are finally both in the mood for sex—and what happens? You get into a fight. The cause is almost impossible to pinpoint, but the effect is: no sex. No doubt there are a few of those sneaky, often unconscious she-demons at work here, awakened by the increase in sexual energy and now doing their little "Rumpelstilskin dance."

The most common demons are probably the ones who are always droning on in the back of your mind, "You should be ... You ought to ... You can't do that right now ... You should have done this or that long ago!" If you think about it, you can probably find dozens of these sex-hostile lecturers. Identify them, express them in a way that harms neither you nor your partner, and then chase them out, away from your love nest!

GOAL
Physically expressing your internal enemies of love so that you don't have to use your strength to keep them in check and their energy doesn't disrupt your love nest.

TIME AND EXTERNAL PREPARATIONS
Five to ten minutes before an erotic encounter, a massage, or a ritual. It's a good idea to have a room big enough for dance and movement, without breakable objects, possibly with drum music playing in the background.

STEP BY STEP
* Stand up straight and close your eyes for a moment.

* Concentrate on all your so-called negative (that is, disruptive) feelings and thoughts, even if they're not as vehemently obvious as they were just yesterday. These include negative thoughts about yourself, about your partner, about your relationship, about sex, and about life in general. Breathe deeply and increase your awareness of these thoughts, even if it feels unpleasant.

✳ Imagine that all of these thoughts and feelings are like small or large she-demons within you, demons that want to be noticed and that strive for expression. Then express them—press them out of you with movements, sounds, grimaces, etc. Allow yourself to make ugly twitching motions, squealing or grinding noises, horrible faces. Seek the extreme and express it. Dance the dance of the she-demons within you.

✳ Some demons give in quickly as soon as they are allowed to rage a little. Others are more persistent. Tell these that they need to calm down and that you'd like to be in a "demon-free zone" right now. After all, your conscious self is the authority of the hour, not the old, distressing ghosts of earlier times. Remind yourself that these she-demons are usually based on outdated patterns, and that you have the option to pay attention to them or send them away.

✳ If the she-demons provide you with important information, don't discard the thoughts; instead, pack them into that famous five-star freezer in your imaginary refrigerator, the one standing next to your love nest that can keep your thoughts fresh until the next day. It is, however, recommended that in due course you really do "take them out" and think them through, so they don't pile up and cause your refrigerator to explode one day—maybe right when you're totally relaxed, just about to concentrate on your new lover in the here and now.

CREATIVE WAYS TO DEAL WITH STUMBLING BLOCKS

The principle "Prevention is better than drilling" (as one might hear at the dentist's office) counts here, too; it's much better to clear up unfinished things—misunderstandings, conflicts, and unconscious sex-hostile norms—than to let yourself be tortured with persistent thoughts that "drill" into you during love games. Prevention, however, is never 100 percent effective, so make an effort to express (literally, to press out) whatever you can, and be generous with yourself if some things continue to "stick"! You'll always have more chances to drive out your she-demons. Also, refresh your memory by reviewing the section "Smart Ways to Manage Distractions" (Chapter 3, page 53).

VARIATIONS AND SUGGESTIONS

You can do this dance of the demons as a couple, too, as preparation for a love game, even if your demons are very different. Express them as much as you can; fight with them, fight with each other until you're exhausted (without hurting each other!)—and at some point you may be able to let this active encounter turn into an aggressive-passionate love game.

If you don't want to merely express your inner demons in order to integrate them, but would rather "drive them out" more effectively, you can try to do that by stopping your dance for a moment, picturing the most active demon as a real person, and asking it what it wants from you. If it has demands you'd rather not fulfill, you will have to negotiate until you've found a solution that speaks for both of you. You can also try, without using words, to discover your own inner need that is hiding behind all the demon's posturing (for example, being recognized in your own way or being important without expectations). If you are able to fulfill this need, you can transform the power of the demon into a force that will help you fulfill your deepest desires.

🐚 Exercise 23: Cleaning out your overflowing love nest

Whenever two lovers cuddle, neck, kiss, play, arouse each other, or passionately throw themselves at each other, thinking that they are alone, this is seldom the case. Often, their love nest is filled with their (inner) parents preaching their own ideas about love and sex, an unforgotten pastor droning on with his pleasure-phobic rants from the pulpit, an earlier teacher croaking out her moralizing warnings. Even a big futon can quickly be filled up that way! Let's empty out the love nest!

GOAL

Identifying internalized authorities and the experiences associated with them, and internally distancing yourself from them.

TIME AND EXTERNAL PREPARATIONS

About five minutes before an erotic encounter.

STEP BY STEP

* ✳ Imagine earlier, or maybe even current, authority figures who have sex-hostile ideas, sayings, or attitudes.

* ✳ If it's important for you, go ahead and say their names.

* ✳ Then open the door and throw them out with a powerful exhalation or a roar of "Get out!"

* ✳ Repeat this until a feeling of relief develops and you have the inner certainty that you alone (or both of you) decide what can and should happen in this love nest.

CREATIVE WAYS TO DEAL WITH STUMBLING BLOCKS

You can, of course, take on your earlier victim role with these earlier authorities and make room for the feelings that accompany that role. However, it is better to save this posture for situations (i.e., conversations with friends or in therapy) in which this side of you will get more attention and you can work on the problems connected with it. For the purposes of this exercise you should consider these guests uninvited, and you should just throw them out without being sensitive and trying to understand them. If you give these intruders attention now, their power grows and you expend energy that you could be using to create new love games.

VARIATIONS AND SUGGESTIONS

This game, too, works wonderfully with two people and can even strengthen you in creating healthy boundaries.

If the uninvited guests are not particularly clear and strong, it may be enough to symbolically place a bowl of rice outside the door for them, to open the door and invite them to enjoy the rice outside, and then to close the door again. This only works, however, if they have not yet gotten too loud and shameless. (I would advise against eating that rice later.)

🍵 Exercise 24: Groaning yoni and laughing belly

This is a good-mood game that is just as strengthening as it is amusing. It doesn't need to be taken seriously, and it allows us to laugh hysterically for a change.

GOAL

Improving your expression of fun and pleasure. By artificially expressing erotic desire, you gradually activate desire's inherent qualities and the ways they are expressed. This way, the hysterically breathed "false tones" can become a real expression of feeling, one in which much of what we have been hiding out of shame or embarrassment comes to the surface.

TIME AND EXTERNAL PREPARATIONS

Two segments of five minutes each, and a couple of minutes of silence afterward.

STEP BY STEP

* Sit or lie down and lay a hand on your yoni (or your mons veneris, if you don't have very long arms).

* Close your eyes and imagine that your yoni is in a state of utmost pleasure and needs to express it.

* Give your yoni a voice, and breathe out sounds of desire: groan, scream, whimper, jubilate, or growl pleasurably. Try out every possible variation and observe how these artificially created sounds feel within you. Exaggerate all the sounds, support them with your breath and movements, become extreme and abandoned. Let all the sounds rush through you like waves, filling up the room around you.

* After five minutes, let the sounds and movements ebb away, and lay one hand on your belly.

* And then start to laugh. Just like that. Start with a loud laugh, laughing at yourself, at both of you, about the latest joke—whatever. Laugh; be broad and raucous or giggly and gulping. Let your heart jump with joy or your belly heave with the comedy of the situation. Play with every possible kind of laugh, and exaggerate each one as much as possible. Even if some are "false notes," laugh until your whole body is shaking and the room is filled with your sounds. Consider how these sounds feel inside you, but don't concentrate too much on your feelings; instead, focus on how they are expressed.

✳ After another five minutes, let yourself become calmer and notice the changes in you without trying to evaluate them.

CREATIVE WAYS TO DEAL WITH STUMBLING BLOCKS

If feelings of shame or embarrassment come up, don't withdraw in silence; instead, express those feelings in your moaning or laughing.

If a stubborn voice says, "I can't do that on command!" then let another part of you be amused that it does work, somehow, particularly if you don't take your little ego so seriously. Even resistance in the form of boredom, or intellectually tearing apart your pitch, can be dissolved by groaning and laughing.

VARIATIONS AND SUGGESTIONS

As a couple, the greater shyness that exists is usually only there at the beginning; after that, it's often followed by mutual "heating up." Expressing your feelings together gives you inner permission to moan and laugh—that is, to create the forms of expression that most easily bring your feelings of desire and pleasure out of the depths and up to the surface.

🍸 Exercise 25: The courage to show yourself

Since we, as women in a patriarchal culture of dominance, have generally learned to hide our bodies and our histories within ourselves, it can be a valuable experience to find the courage to show more of ourselves in a familiar atmosphere.

GOAL

Losing all feelings of shame and encouraging a realistic view of your own body and your self-respect, as well as obtaining an increased understanding of your own body's history. The goal is also to show yourself in a way that exactly represents how you feel inside. Thus, this striptease can become an exercise in self-love, reflected in a loving gaze.

TIME AND EXTERNAL PREPARATIONS

Two segments of about forty minutes each, as well as a few minutes to exchange thoughts afterward.

STEP BY STEP

✳ First, greet each other with a heart-to-heart embrace. The way this works is that each person first expands and enlivens their own heart chakra with a couple of deep breaths. Then walk toward the other person, slowly and with a straight back, and look at your partner with an open gaze and a full heart, and embrace your partner, letting one hand rest on the other's rear heart chakra (just below the shoulder blades) for a moment. Now give each other a small, honest compliment (sometimes even without words) and carefully free yourself from the embrace.

✳ *If you're the active partner,* while the other person sits comfortably, begin to undress so slowly that you can observe your own feelings while your partner watches you openly and lovingly.

✳ Show yourself, increasingly naked, and meanwhile tell the other person about your relationship to your body, its various parts, and their histories.

✳ *If you're the observing and listening partner,* after about fifteen minutes, give a loving and honest response to what you see, and describe any associations that come to you.

✳ Finally, the one who so bravely showed herself is allowed to make a wish. For example, maybe you want to be spoiled by your partner in order to reinvigorate less vigorous parts or to feel the sensation of being accepted. Feathers or other sensual objects could be used as aids, or you can even use massage oil.

✳ Afterward, switch roles.

CREATIVE WAYS TO DEAL WITH STUMBLING BLOCKS

When you are the active partner, while you are doing the telling, as you investigate pain from old injuries, it may be that you get stuck there, feeling like you are only made up of old hurts, old self-rejection, or old shame. A loving reassurance from the other usually helps you show yourself, yet without any pressure.

VARIATIONS AND SUGGESTIONS

The variation that includes three people often has the advantage that both listeners increase their creativity in terms of positive and honest responses; in this way, the person showing herself has a greater feeling of being accepted. In the spoiling phase, the active partner's reward for having the courage to show herself is not as tied to one person, which makes another kind of self-related pleasure possible (for example, a little "massage in stereo," where the recipient is spoiled simultaneously from both sides).

🦋 Exercise 26: Letting the being in the female lap speak

On the mental-spiritual level of sexual identity, this exercise does what the striptease does on a physical level: It creates more awareness of one's own createdness and thus allows a chance to free oneself from old patterns of self-handicapping or self-rejection. In particular, it deals with the location of our deepest female power: our laps.

GOAL

Giving your innermost sexual self a voice; becoming more aware of your own sexual history and learning to integrate it.

TIME AND EXTERNAL PREPARATIONS

Two or three segments of about twenty minutes each, and the same amount of time afterward for exchanging thoughts about the exercise.

STEP BY STEP

* *If you're the active partner,* wear an open or half-covering sarong (a long skirtcloth, also known as a *pareo*) or sit naked, and stroke a little scented oil on your yoni (caution—only on the outside, or it might sting!). Now lay your hand there and gradually lift the curtain to show your yoni to your partner.

* *If you're the observing partner,* watch while holding one hand on your heart and wearing a soft gaze, and say words of sensual, flowery description and honor for the now-visible lap of your beloved.

* If you're the one doing the showing, lay your hand on your yoni and lend it your voice by reporting, in first-person narrative, on its life with the woman to whom it belongs.

* The other partner listens without interjecting, and gives a loving *and* honest response at the end (only in this combination). Meanwhile, as the active partner, you can show your yoni one more time and perhaps receive further compliments and loving descriptions.

* Afterward, switch roles, and then exchange thoughts about your experiences.

CREATIVE WAYS TO DEAL WITH STUMBLING BLOCKS

Women who have experienced distinct external changes in their labia or other parts of their laps as a result of surgery or giving birth are often shy about showing themselves because they find themselves ugly. Sometimes the only thing that helps here is allowing a few tears and/or expressions of anger over these unwanted changes before you find the courage to carefully present yourself before another's eyes and to open yourself to what comes back to you in looks and words. Usually, the other's loving devotion is felt as a great relief and encouragement.

VARIATIONS AND SUGGESTIONS

You can also do this exercise alone in front of a mirror and give your yoni a "written voice"; that is, one hand rests on your yoni while the other writes down what the yoni would write.

🐦 Exercise 27: The body-map of love

Things you have drawn out in black (or bright colors) on white are usually more firmly implanted in your brain and are therefore more easily accessible when dealing with your awareness of your uniqueness as a woman.

GOAL

Increasing consciousness of the multiplicity of female pleasure centers and of the possibilities for awakening them and joyously observing them.

TIME AND EXTERNAL PREPARATIONS

At least an hour of quiet time and afterward about twenty minutes for an exchange. Paste together pieces of butcher paper or scraps of wrapping paper so they are long enough to fit a life-size outline of a person on them; finger paints or oil pastels are recommended for drawing.

STEP BY STEP

* One person lies down on a piece of paper and has her outline traced by a partner. Then roles are switched.

* Next, each partner finds their own space and lays another piece of paper over the drawing in order to copy the outline, so that each can draw a picture of both the front and the back of the body.

* Now the assignment is to draw in all your erogenous zones on the picture and to rank them with numbers in order to show how you would most like to be pampered for maximal pleasure.

* Taboo zones or "cold zones" can be shaded in a different color.

* "Learning zones" can be cross-hatched.

* Finally, the evaluative exchange with your partner is crucial. The point is not to analyze each other and your body-maps pseudo-psychoanalytically, but to share associations having to do with the body as landscape and with parts of this landscape, and to possibly bring in your own experiences in a supportive way.

CREATIVE WAYS TO DEAL WITH STUMBLING BLOCKS

Some women simply leave parts of their bodies blank because they have never experienced how this body part feels when it is filled with sexual energy. This can lead to expressions of self-rejection. It sometimes helps to remember that you can fill in the empty zones as "learning zones"—areas where you might use your breathing to distribute energy more strongly, so that you can have pleasurable experiences in those areas as well.

Sometimes the drawing is not differentiated enough to produce an informative picture. Here it may help to take more time to investigate yourself more closely, with self-love, and then to share more detailed or contextually different erotic-sexual responses that individual body parts experience when given special attention. Also, the saying holds true here: Even the smallest puddle can reflect the sky.

VARIATIONS AND SUGGESTIONS

If the two partners join with another couple for later exchanges, there sometimes develops a stable square (quadrangle) in which interviews about intimate stimuli and desires are made possible, and creative new sex ideas can be born.

🍃 Exercise 28: Sexual menu

As an XXL woman who also likes to revel in good food, I was very happy about the book *Aphrodite: A Feast for the Senses,* by Isabel Allende. In it, she reports on her unwillingness to separate good food from good sex. I personally find that the principles of preparing a good meal and good lovemaking abilities are similar. This inspired me to create this exercise, which is intended to creatively expand our wishes and possibilities, and to forge plans to make them a reality.

GOAL
Reveling in wishes and fantasized possibilities, with the option to playfully make them real.

TIME AND EXTERNAL PREPARATIONS
At least an hour. Have various index cards and pens handy.

STEP BY STEP
* Each person takes about a quarter of an hour to create three lists on three different index cards. List all the "makers" of pleasure (mouth, fingers, etc.); all the activities of pleasure (stroking, kissing, biting, etc.); and all the recipients of pleasure (clitoris, anus, mouth, etc.).

* You can then exchange lists. You may, of course, "copy" from the other person if they've listed something that seems pleasurable to you.

* Then you both discuss which activities listed by either partner are anatomically and acrobatically possible for the enjoyer, and which might be desirable.

* After that, each of you retreat to your own space and use another, possibly bigger, index card to put together a sexual menu of the things you would most like to enjoy right now. For example, you

could write down the ambiance you'd most like to have, which aperitif you'd prefer, what should make up the appetizer list, and the entrées, all the way up to dessert. Be sure to include spices, drinks, and the presentation as well as the dinner music. You can even specify the amount of time to be spent on each course and the participants you would like to include in your love feast. Any ideas that are basically achievable, that are technically and acrobatically performable, and that don't damage your partner's dignity are welcome here.

✳ From this menu, you can make up a wish list that you might, for example, hand over to your partner before your next birthday. You should indicate that this is not a firm plan, but instead a collection of pleasurable ideas, suggestions for expanding and playfully satisfying your mutual desires.

✳ When handing over the wish list, it is important to see it as a present to your partner—a present of openness, expressed through the precise description of your own wishes. It represents taking responsibility for your own needs rather than making the other person try to guess them (yet again).

CREATIVE WAYS TO DEAL WITH STUMBLING BLOCKS
Many women have trouble with classic obstacle phrases like "That's not going to work!" or "My partner definitely doesn't want to do that!" It may be that some desires really don't work out within a relationship or in a particular situation. However, there are some helpful phrases to remember, like "Learn by playing" and "Practice makes perfect."

VARIATIONS AND SUGGESTIONS
If these kinds of wish lists tend to increase performance pressure and fear of failure, it is sometimes worthwhile just to exchange lists and talk about them without trying to make them a reality. Doing so may create the possibility of talking about your sexual preferences and about potential pleasure variations.

🐚 *Exercise 29: Body painting from back to front, via the heart*

Here, in contrast to the "body-map of love," qualities and emotional states are drawn directly on the body, temporarily making it easier to identify with them.

GOAL
Accepting your own body as well as transforming past injuries.

TIME AND EXTERNAL PREPARATIONS
At least an hour for each partner, plus time for an exchange afterward—altogether about two and a half hours. You need a color-safe cloth that is placed on top of a comfortable mattress, hypoallergenic paints, and two good-sized mirrors. It's useful to have some coarse sea salt and also a mixture of cornmeal and cream to get the paint out of your pores afterward.

STEP BY STEP
  * Sit across from each other with your eyes closed, and think about which of *your own* qualities (not your partner's!) stand in the way of pleasurable sexuality—which parts of yourself, in other words, you would gradually like to leave behind. Then decide which of your qualities could be helpful for the growth and development of your sexual pleasure—that is, which qualities you would like to strengthen in the future.

  * Next, discuss with your partner these groups of qualities and express how you would like to have them painted on your body— even if the painter follows her own creativity in the end.

  * *If you're the painter,* your partner now lies down on her belly. Begin to paint on your partner's back all the qualities your partner would like to leave behind. After a short pause to let the paint dry, your partner rolls over and you paint her front side with all the qualities she wants to develop in the future.

  * *If you're the one being painted,* once the colors have dried, look at yourself, both front and back, in two large, opposed mirrors, and give the painter some brief feedback. After a short period of

silence and meditation on how the qualities painted on your back make you feel, mentally switch over to the qualities on your front side, the ones you want to develop, and attempt to identify strongly with them, as though you were only made up of these qualities.

✳ Now begin to do a "dance of the future qualities." Feel them out, show them to your partner through movement, and receive an honest compliment on these qualities and the possibility of developing them further.

✳ Now switch roles.

✳ Afterward, do a dance together, a combining of the past and the future in the present.

✳ Finally, discuss the transformation of the past into the future and of apathy into desire.

CREATIVE WAYS TO DEAL WITH STUMBLING BLOCKS

If a woman feels too naked to show herself comfortably and fearlessly, even with body paint, it's a good idea for her to take time alone in front of the mirror and to show the other person only as much as she wants to. (Throwing a sarong or a blanket around yourself is no problem once the paint has dried.)

VARIATIONS AND SUGGESTIONS

As long as it doesn't create any undue pressure, each partner can have photos taken of their front and back so they can remind themselves of the exercise later, even after the paint has been washed off.

ℳ Exercise 30: Dance of the hands

This playful exercise is an excellent transitional ritual from the activeness of everyday occurrences to a sensitive contact with each other. Besides, this is a game of boundaries and the many ways you can expand them. The rules for our meadow of pleasure are the same as they are for any garden: The number of flowers, not the fence, is what's important.

GOAL

A sensitive encounter, and finding many ways of vibrating in tune with each other.

TIME AND EXTERNAL PREPARATIONS

About thirty minutes, and ten minutes to exchange thoughts. Select appealing music to accompany the exercise.

STEP BY STEP

* Stand or squat in front of each other, in such a way that you can easily touch each other's hands with your arms bent.

* Slowly move your palms toward each other, and very gently touch fingertips. Now close your eyes.

* In time with quiet music, gently move your fingers together. Each of you concentrate on your own feelings during this contact, on the process of leading and following, and on the energy that now flows between you and your partner.

* Next, play somewhat stronger, more rhythmic music, while both of you begin to move your fingertips playfully, exploring, teasing, tickling, and feeling the hands that you are feeling for the first time or the familiar hands that you are rediscovering.

* Now your whole hands touch. Begin to make stronger motions that can become more aggressive or even become little power plays—but without hurting each other.

* The more aggressive movements become broader, more energetic motions that are more room-grabbing than aggressive; the nonverbally assigned roles of leader and follower are more clearly lived out and can always be exchanged.

* After reaching an energetic high point, the movements grow smaller, more delicate, and gentler to the touch. Each of you concentrates on the image of your arms and hands as wings of the heart, using your hands to touch the other's heart and receiving a heartfelt touch from the other.

* After a few farewell gestures, slowly let go of each other's hands.

✳ Each of you clasps your own hands together and takes a few moments to meditate.

✳ Finally, discuss the encounter.

CREATIVE WAYS TO DEAL WITH STUMBLING BLOCKS
For some, suddenly surfacing feelings of aggression, longing, or eroticism are frightening; they may try to minimize these feelings by "laughing them off." If you have this experience, you can make the feelings "bearable" by concentrating on expressing them exclusively with your fingers and hands.

🖋 Exercise 31: The chakra wave

The chakra wave is another step in preparing to play freely with your sexual energy; it not only "blows through" the individual chakras, but also charges them up more strongly. This purification process helps sexual energy flow through you without hindrance and helps you feel how it is colored by each chakra's individual qualities. Thus, you can continue to flow with all the colors in you, and maybe you can even pour yourself out into the colorful sea of oceanic feelings. To familiarize yourself with the concept of chakras, before you begin the exercise you might want to review "A Short Lesson on the Chakras" in Chapter 2, page 42.

GOAL
Cleaning and charging the individual chakra funnels, freeing them up for playing with sexual energy.

TIME AND EXTERNAL PREPARATIONS
About twenty minutes per partner, sitting or standing.

STEP BY STEP
    ✳ Begin with the heart-to-heart embrace (see Exercise 25, "The courage to show yourself").

    ✳ Once you both feel comfortable and relaxed, sit down so that the "breather" (the one doing the active breathing) is seated in front of the companion, who is also comfortably seated, with legs spread, or squatting. The breather's legs may be crossed. Briefly tune in to each other.

✳ *If you're the companion,* lay your hands around the breather in such a way that they touch her yoni (either the perineum as the outer gate or at least the mons veneris). Use your fingertips to tap on it a couple of times, as if to awaken this part of the body.

✳ *If you're the breather,* now breathe deeply, concentrating the whole of your inhalations and exhalations on your root chakra. Breathe so powerfully that you take in more energy than you need. In this way, you charge up the chakra. Once the root chakra has been sufficiently charged, all kinds of feelings connected with it may come up. Now it is your job to push all of these feelings out using sounds, movements, and other forms of expression, thus recharging your chakra again and again with powerful breaths.

✳ *If you're the companion,* leave one hand on your partner's yoni and now move your other hand up the other chakras one by one, gently tapping on the appropriate spot or letting your hand rest there, while the breather charges up all the chakras, one after the other, in order to express the feelings that develop there. (If you're practicing alone, you can leave one hand on your yoni and briefly touch your other chakras; however, if you're expressing more emotions, your hands will probably be all over the place, everywhere *but* your chakras. Nevertheless, with each transition you can return to the appropriate chakra, touching it briefly.)

✳ As the breather, you may find that you need less powerful breaths to charge up the higher chakras and that the feelings connected with the higher chakras may also be different from the lower chakras' more slowly vibrating energy forms (e.g., the muffled growling heard from the belly region). In any case, the real feelings that come up, bound to each chakra in this moment, are more important than any preconceived ideas.

✳ Once you have reached the crown chakra, the breather emphatically breathes through the whole system, between root and crown chakra, one more time. In doing so, imagine that you are breathing fire from your lap, from bottom to top, out beyond yourself; your exhalation trickles back down onto you, light as a feather.

✳ Then, breather, lean back into your companion's arms and relax for a moment before you lie down beside each other and discuss your experiences.

✳ Afterward, switch roles.

CREATIVE WAYS TO DEAL WITH STUMBLING BLOCKS

Some companions put enormous effort into trying not to move, which might disrupt the breather's process, or into leaving one hand on the root chakra even if they have short arms. Instead, the companion should follow a basic rule of thumb: It's better to readjust your position or let go of one hand than to get a cramp and transfer your tension to your partner.

Sometimes the companion's hand is irritatingly off center or their touch is too forceful or too weak or just not pleasant at the moment. If this is the case, it's a good idea to lovingly correct her and tell her what would better support your process.

Some breathers have so many pictures and phrases about chakras in their heads that they hardly recognize their inner reality or judge it to be "wrong" or "inappropriate." If this happens to you, focus on your quality of childlike curiosity, the one that wants to find out about everything and learn about nature's magic. (For example, imagine that you are a little girl with no learned shame or fear. For this child, it's normal to investigate every orifice, to look at each one with amazement, and to want to know what can come out of or go into it.)

Some breathers want to spend more time on one chakra and skip another; you can do that if you like, but sometimes it's better not to get wrapped up in the potentially difficult feelings of one chakra. Instead, you should keep going, and then repeat the exercise a week later, maybe even twice, in order to express any traumas or difficult feelings "in installments."

If sitting one behind the other is too hard for either of you, the breather can instead stand or lie down while the companion either sits by her side or stands behind her and touches her chakras one at a time.

Some companions want to do a good job of supporting the breather, and they end up breathing so loudly or strongly that the breather loses her own rhythm. If as the companion you want to support the expression of emotions, you can breathe along, but you should let the breather take the lead.

VARIATIONS AND SUGGESTIONS

Here is one more suggestion for how to use music to energetically support the (not uncomplicated!) chakra wave. (This goes for the "Fire-breathing orgasm" as well, Exercise 46.) More details on the music listed below can be found in the Resources section.

❋ MUSIC TO GO WITH THE CHAKRA WAVE

Chakra connections		Music
I	root	*Totem* (track 1)
I → II	root → navel	*La Luna* (track 2)
I → III	root → solar plexus	*La Luna* (track 1)
II → III	navel → solar plexus	*Feet in the Soil* (track 5)
II → IV	navel → heart	*Feet in the Soil* (track 6)
III → IV	solar plexus → heart	*Return to the Goddess* (track 6)
III → V	solar plexus → larynx	*Shepherd Moons* (track 2)
IV → V	heart → larynx	*Hidden Waters* (track 5)
IV → VI	heart → third eye	*Shekhina* (track 3)
V → VI	larynx → third eye	*Hidden Waters* (track 2)
V → VII	larynx → crown	*Shekhina* (track 5)
VI → VII	third eye → crown	*From Source to Sea* (tracks 1, 3)
VII	crown	*Im Garten der Liebe* (In the Garden of Love; track 4)
VII → I	crown → root	*Return to the Goddess* (tracks 1, 2)
Silence! ...		
Resurfacing/Emerging		*Ancient Mother* (tracks 2, 4)

After the chakra wave, the breather can go into the "butterfly" (see "Sexual breathing," Exercise 15) while the companion sits behind you and holds your outstretched hands.

After a few wing movements of the well-ventilated butterfly's body, loins and souls usually become as soft as butter in the morning sun. Then, as the breather, you can open your eyes and see that your companion is giving you a little smile. If it is honestly possible, as the breather, now lying relaxed, you can whisper or breathe out a "yes!": a yes to your companion on this journey through the chakras; a yes to the process undertaken together; a yes to a possibly deepened trust; and then a *"Yesss!"* to yourself—to your desire, your pain, your anger, your exhaustion, and your sense of vitality as you are now aware of it. Then close your eyes one more time and imagine that the yes is filling your whole body with each inhalation and exhalation. Stretch out the yes even further: It can become a yes to all women, a yes to all the processes of animate nature, a yes to being tied in to the world.

🐚 Exercise 32: Swinging into a state of melting

The point of this game, which you play first by yourself and then together with another person, is to make freeing motions with your pelvis.

GOAL
Physically preparing yourself for pelvic motions and encounters that can then be used in harmony as a couple.

TIME AND EXTERNAL PREPARATIONS
Approximately forty-five minutes. Lovers who are experienced with each other can agree to make it open-ended. I'd recommend using a low, firm cushion or, for those with knee problems, a higher firm cushion. And be sure to change positions occasionally. You will also need two tennis balls.

STEP BY STEP
First, for you alone

* *Make your pelvis flexible:* Sit up straight, close your eyes, and move your pelvis forward as you breathe out and backward as you breathe in. Once you have grown accustomed to this motion, include your whole spine, so that your upper body moves along passively.

* *Loosening up with a rocking motion while sitting:* Sit so that you can feel your sitting bones, and straighten yourself from there all the way up to your crown. Then rotate your upper body in such a way that you massage the tissue around your sit bones. Now imagine that you can "walk" on your sit bones, and slowly move forward in this way.

* *Loosening up with tennis balls:* Sit down with one tennis ball under each buttock, and forcefully breathe out through those points of contact. Then lie down, having put the two tennis balls into a sock so that they stay together. Place the tennis balls under your buttocks, in about the middle, and move them up along the muscles on either side of your spine, inch by inch, pausing for a few seconds each time. During these pauses, imagine breathing out through the tennis balls, and make sounds—especially wherever you feel painful tension. Then sit up again, cross your legs, and place a tennis ball under your perineum; breathe in while pumping your PC muscle, imagine the inner flute (see Exercise 16), and gently breathe out. (If this is too uncomfortable, don't bother; this isn't a book for would-be masochists. If you feel moderate or aching pain, imagine breathing through the tennis ball until the pain turns into warmth or a feeling of wideness.)

* Share these experiences, which may take some getting used to, with the other person (including the sounds you make when pressure is placed on your tense spots).

Then, together

* Stand up, one partner behind the other. The person in back begins to make pelvic motions forward, then to the side, and then backward while the other follows her lead. Then the partner in front leads, and the one in back follows.

* Next, contract your PC muscle with every backward pelvic motion and relax it with every forward pelvic motion.

* Then stand across from each other and close your eyes. Each of you then makes your own pelvic movements, occasionally contract-

ing the PC muscle. Then open your eyes and decide which person will lead. If you're the leader, move your pelvis forward as you exhale and backward as you inhale. The other partner does the same, following the leader's rhythm.

* Then the first partner continues rocking the pelvis and the other breathes in when the first partner breathes out, and vice versa.

* Play with different ways of breathing for a while, breathing parallel or opposite each other while moving your pelvic bones. Allow yourselves to observe the differences in your feelings. Afterward, each of you take back your own energy, close your eyes to meditate for a moment, and then sit down for a verbal exchange.

CREATIVE WAYS TO DEAL WITH STUMBLING BLOCKS
Some people feel pressured by the different breathing possibilities or use the space for smaller or larger power games. It's important to experiment with the principle of trial and error and to use errors as an impulse for further attempts.

Some want to be technically perfect and end up confused. This confusion can often be resolved by leaving yourself time to feel, by looking at the other person and their movements, or even by deciding to forget all the instructions and breathing suggestions and just playing with each other.

🐟 Exercise 33: The yab-yum love position

This exercise playfully helps improve your attitude toward breathing together. In conjunction with the sexual heat before or instead of orgasmic ecstasy or even with the exhausted delirium afterward, this position helps steer the fire of love through the chakras and simultaneously fuses one partner to the other person's chakras.

GOAL
Playing with lively, creative, nonverbal communication on the "lower level" of the body, where fire energy melts into a wide lava flow and can be guided through the chakras in all directions by your breathing.

TIME AND EXTERNAL PREPARATIONS
About an hour.

STEP BY STEP

* Stand belly-to-belly with your partner, and try to breathe alternately, using belly breathing only. When inhaling, one of you fills your belly while the other breathes out and flattens theirs; when exhaling, the first partner then flattens their belly while the other expands their own. If the alternate breathing works well as a belly-breathing technique, the two of you can look at each other and gradually release yourselves from the close physical contact without changing your alternate breathing.

* Now stand about two yards apart and kick an imaginary ball back and forth. You can catch and bounce the ball with your bellies, hips, feet, heads, etc. What is important is that you catch or return the ball immediately so that an exchange develops. Bring that wild girl back out of your body's memory.

* Next, sit across from each other in the heart-to-heart greeting (see Exercise 25), without touching, and play a little with the camel ride and sexual breathing until each of you is comfortably rocking by yourself.

* Now make eye contact, and move closer to each other by sitting close together with your thighs overlapping. Only when the intimacy between you feels right does one sit down in the other's lap (yab-yum; see Figure 5 on page 137). It is important for both to sit up straight and not lean in either direction. You can support yourselves with your hands on the other's back (i.e., on the rear heart chakra and the rear navel chakra), so that the energy can flow upward or to the other's chakra more easily. There are many ways to enjoy the energy flow in the yab-yum position, so play with the pelvic rocking motion, with your PC muscle, and with your sexual breathing. You can do this in tandem or alternately. When breathing alternately, the bottom partner largely determines the rhythm, but she coordinates with the partner on top. For the pelvic rocking

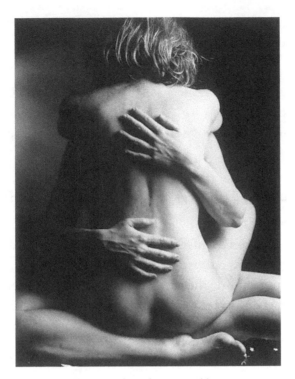

Figure 5. The yab-yum position.

motion, there is the energetic parallel kick (the strength of the movement increases exponentially) or the harmonizing alternating rocking (like a slow, calming camel ride over gentle sand dunes). Try them out to see which is most pleasurable for both of you at the moment.

CREATIVE WAYS TO DEAL WITH STUMBLING BLOCKS

If one partner is too heavy for the other, the heavier one can place a pillow underneath herself or himself when on top, so that the upper legs exert less pressure. If neither is very flexible in the pelvic region, you can try this exercise on a chair. If both tend toward muscle cramps, you can change positions frequently.

Some think they have to "master" the yab-yum position right away. Please remember that this position is usually the product of lengthy practice in sitting poses, a practice that cannot be skipped entirely. So allow yourself to play and experiment, and to feel the effects of different sitting positions on your body.

VARIATIONS AND SUGGESTIONS
Rather than having someone's legs fall asleep or thigh muscles cramp up, you can always sit with your legs draped over each other's. Again, remember: Allow as much variation as necessary and as little disruption as possible.

🕊 *Exercise 34: Submission without ifs, ands, or buts*

This game can be a wonderful lead-in to a love game as well as an excellent ending. In addition, this exercise can create feelings of loving affection and devotion without requiring the participants to be love partners, and without the exercise having to be a love game in the narrower sexual sense.

GOAL
Becoming softer and more receptive in order to give in to loving touches and gazes.

TIME AND EXTERNAL PREPARATIONS
About an hour. You need a mat big enough for two and a large towel or sheet that you don't mind getting stained with oil. For clothing, use a sarong or a cloth around the hips.

STEP BY STEP
   * Stand across from each other and begin with a variation on the heart-to-heart greeting. Cross both hands over your own heart, consciously breathe into them a few times, then open your hands and arms wide, imagining that the energy in your heart is growing as wide as your arms and is able to envelop the other person. Then encircle each other with your arms so that your breasts are touching, and linger in this tender embrace for a moment.

   * Now one of you—whom I will call the rose—begins to show yourself clearly and seductively in your sarong or some other easily removable outfit. At the same time, the other—whom I will call

the orchid—watches with the eyes of the heart. After exchanging a small compliment, switch roles.

✳ Next, the rose carefully begins to remove the orchid's sarong, and the orchid does the same to the rose. Both begin a little dance of veiling and unveiling with the cloths, each holding the other's piece of clothing.

✳ After this, sit or squat across from each other and gradually begin to activate your inner wildness, moving together in a passionate-wild way (see also "Dance of the hands," Exercise 30, or "Dance of the she-demons," Exercise 22).

✳ As you allow your contact to grow gentler again, both of you "vibrate" with wave breathing (that is, sexual breathing combined with pumping the PC muscle and rocking the pelvis; see Exercise 50). First do this on your own, separately, then in rhythm with one other. (You can also use the yab-yum position.)

✳ Now the rose begins to rub sesame or olive oil on the orchid. If you're the orchid, you can be seated in the rose's lap or between her legs, leaning back, or you can assume the yab-yum position to have your back anointed. It is important for the orchid to give in more and more to the hands of the rose, while, at the same time, maintaining your own wave motions.

✳ Now, switch roles. The rose is given the same pleasurable treatment.

✳ Then both of you stretch your limbs and return to the yab-yum position. Imagine you are fusing together to become one sensual flower, and again begin the wave motion, simultaneously rocking with your hips and passively moving your backs in a wave pattern.

✳ The wave motion grows softer and calmer, and regular alternate breathing and PC pumping can be added to it.

✳ At the end it may be that your wave motions are so subtle that they are invisible from the outside. But inside, you may feel a gentle rippling, an intimate sense of peace—or even the desire to move more vigorously again. There are no rules, just a mutual arrangement of your desires.

CREATIVE WAYS TO DEAL WITH STUMBLING BLOCKS
If the yab-yum gets too uncomfortable for the partner on the bottom, you can sit facing each other with your upper legs laid over each other's, and you can switch off occasionally so that no one feels strained and gets distracted.

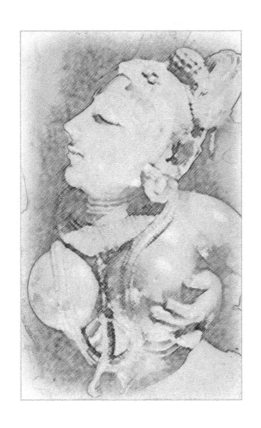

≈ CHAPTER 7 ≈

Massages That Have
What It Takes

*O*f the following massages, the first one serves as a bit of an intro-
ductory exercise. From the breast massage onwards, the exercises
are increasingly about awakening and subtly spreading erotic-sexual energy
into your heart, as the center of your love for yourself and the world, and
to the other chakras, in order to stimulate and nourish them and to transform the respective feelings in them. By *transform* I mean to turn all feelings and sensations into pure life energy by bringing into them the
awareness of the breath, by expressing them and letting them live, by letting them be and thus letting them go again.

Exercise 35: Pressing instead of talking

Sometimes all this "talking about it" causes us to lose sight of the actual
experience. And yet a pleasure companion can't necessarily sense what the
recipient of her massages wants at a particular moment. That's why it's a
good idea to develop a language without too many words that makes it
easy for both parties to get back to the level of sensing and feeling.

This massage can get more sensual and erotic than is spelled out here
in words. The extent to which this is possible depends on each encounter,
on the feelings of both partners, and on their courage.

GOAL
Practicing active passivity and enjoyable silence without completely giving
up responsibility for yourself.

TIME AND EXTERNAL PREPARATIONS
Two segments of thirty minutes each, plus a little time to discuss afterward. You need a mat and a nice blanket; toys and other objects for sensual-erotic pleasures.

STEP BY STEP
  * *If you're the pleasure companion,* first adapt to the breathing of
    the person lying in front of you, and allow yourself to play with
    the recipient's body intuitively, however you feel is right. You can
    try out anything you want as long as you pay attention to the
    recipient and react promptly to her signals.

✳ *If you're the enjoyer,* you can lie down first on your stomach, then on your back on a mat covered with a nice-looking blanket or sheet. Breathe deeply and imagine that your pores are taking in all that is good; with a deep breath, draw the goodness in even deeper. Everything you don't like is sent back out as you breathe out. In order to make it clear what you want, you can arrange something like the following with your companion ahead of time: Give a signal with your left hand when you like something and with your right if you want it to stop. That way you don't have to say a word, and you can give in to your sounds and your breathing and your feelings without having to distract yourself from the input that lets the massage be pleasurable for you. What is important, in the case of an unpleasant touch, is that you briefly express any anger that might come up but don't get stuck on that feeling; instead, you must try to take in the next touch.

✳ After a while, a second phase begins. The recipient further expresses her feelings with short instructions, like "harder," "softer," "faster," "slower," etc.

✳ After starting the massage with hand contact, the pleasure companion can continue with other objects or body parts like

— ostrich feathers or even a fan made of feathers

— a leather glove in combination with a satin one

— flowers or plants without thorns or sharp stems

— wooden massage balls or rollers

— metal wheels for gently poking the skin (the housewife's version: pastry wheels)

— long hair and fingernails; for some, buzz cuts can be erotic

— vibrators with various attachments

— nubby latex pillows or latex gloves with lubricant

— strings of pearls and other skin-friendly jewelry

— breasts, lips, and other body parts good for stroking

CREATIVE WAYS TO DEAL WITH STUMBLING BLOCKS
As the companion, any stress you may feel about whether you are doing the exercise "right" can usually be resolved if both parties are constantly in attentive, nonverbal contact with each other.

VARIATIONS AND SUGGESTIONS
As the recipient, so that you don't have to waste too many words in conveying your wishes, you can, for example, take your companion's hand and lead it, or demonstrate a touch you'd like to feel, placing your hand on your companion's back.

Exercise 36: Breast massage for the sensual, self-sufficient woman

Our breasts are not just outer symbols of femininity; they are also the hills and sometimes even the wings beneath which our hearts beat, and they are excellent receptors and givers of eroticism—as long as they are given plenty of attention, awakened, and pampered. In addition, the kundalini force as a subtle sexual force (see page 30) is most easily awakened in us women when the nipples are stimulated. (See also "Kundalini massage," Exercise 39.)

GOAL
Lovingly touching the breasts, since these outer features of womanhood can, beyond patriarchal norms of beauty, create an inner feeling of your own female identity and beauty. In addition, daily stroking and massaging of your breasts can stimulate hormone production; in this way, you can lessen menstrual pains, regulate your cycle (even partially stop it, if desired), and improve your awareness of each phase of the cycle.

TIME AND EXTERNAL PREPARATIONS
About five minutes, daily if you like.

STEP BY STEP
As preparation for the breast massage, several Taoist breast-energy exercises have proven to be very helpful:

Cooling off when too much energy has (subjectively) developed

("Too much energy" might be felt as pain, pressure, or inner unease.)

* Take the basic classic bioenergetic stance (feet hip-width apart and flat on the ground, knees slightly bent, pelvis in middle position between front and back, spine straightened, head held high and straight, shoulders lowered).

* While breathing in, bring your arms up along your sides, reaching above your head.

* Then turn your palms toward the earth, holding them above your head; place your right hand on top of your left.

* As you breathe out, guide your hands slowly downward with a loud "Heeeeeeee!" and lead the heat out of your upper body through your legs into the ground.

Finding relief from a feeling of emotional "fullness"

When your heart is filled with grief or pain or frustration, these feelings overflow and are stored in the breasts. By relieving and cleansing the breasts, you can relieve your heart, too.

* Take the basic bioenergetic stance and close your eyes.

* Imagine that you are breathing in golden light through your third eye (see "A Short Lesson on the Chakras" in Chapter 2, page 42).

* Breathe this light from the third eye into your breasts and fill them with it.

* As you breathe out, guide everything that is burdensome and heavy through your legs and feet, out of your body, and into the earth. The earth has the power to transform your energy into pure earth-fire.

* To support yourself, you can use your hands to brush the energy out of your breasts and down into the earth.

Air in the breast

* Take the basic bioenergetic stance and close your eyes.

✳ With your breathing and your concentration, create a connection with your breasts so that you are able to feel them in all their softness, openness, or even in their need for protection.

✳ Try to say a quiet little inner "yes!" to them. If this seems too hard, hum to them a little bit.

✳ While breathing, charge your breasts with as much energy as you find comfortable.

✳ With your imagination, lend this energy a quality that could be good for your breasts—for example, the golden light of the rising sun or the blue sky or a green tree or a sparkling jewel—or simply whatever might occur to you.

✳ If the image is something destructive, send it out into the air through your solar plexus with a hefty exhalation, and breathe pure breath-energy back into your breasts.

✳ Finally, lay both hands on your breasts, and breathe very slowly and calmly until the breath-energy fills your breasts, overflows, and spreads out through your whole body.

Breast massage

✳ Take the basic stance. (You could also do this while sitting, lying down, or squatting.)

✳ Cup both hands under your breasts like a "natural bra," and feel their weight.

✳ Then concentrate your breathing on the contents of your hands, and give yourself and your breasts a little present: As you concentrate on them, draw the corners of your mouth up slowly toward your ears—and smile at them. Smile even if it's a sad or a shy smile.

✳ Then move your hands slowly in a circular motion around your breasts (even if the outer parts are no longer present in "hill" form)—thoughtfully, consciously, and as tenderly or forcefully as you like.

✳ Massage your breasts in a circle about thirty or forty times, and try both directions: The movement from the middle of the breast upward and out has a spreading, stretching effect, and from the bottom inward a concentrating and collecting one. Probably, you will quickly find your favorite direction. Stick with it. (If you use oil in your massage, use rose oil, mix your own breast massage oil, or find a specially premixed oil. This associates a pleasant smell with the positive stimulation of your breast tissue or your heart chakra.)

✳ Then play around a little; massage more firmly or gently, slower or faster, more broadly or just around your nipples.

✳ You can also lay both hands on your breasts, using gentle pressure, and use your breasts to massage your ribcage.

✳ Repeat only what really feels good.

✳ Now let your movements grow softer, and let your circles grow smaller, until finally you gently circle around your nipples and caress them in the most arousing way. Vibrate them, twist them, knead them, or dance on them, circling and bouncing on them with a gentle, featherlike touch or with strong and sharp stroking from fingernails.

✳ Close with the cupped position and an inner smile to your breasts, or by crossing your hands over your heart chakra, reminding yourself of the connection between heart and breast.

CREATIVE WAYS TO DEAL WITH STUMBLING BLOCKS

If you have had to give up a lot of tissue from one or both breasts as a result of breast surgery, concentrate less on their weight than on the skin contact between your breasts and your hands. Hold yourself tenderly and firmly, close your eyes, and feel how you are holding yourself. Remind yourself that externally amputated breasts (just like our other parts) remain energetically present (their aura waves are even measurable) if you retain them as part of your body image and empower them with your mental concentration.

Uncertainty and alienation from their own bodies causes some women to initially execute this exercise quite "technically." If this is the case with you, remind yourself that with every caress you are touching yourself as a woman. Then your massage will have a deeper sense of awareness.

Some women fall back into old judgment patterns with the first touches ("My breasts are too small, too big, saggy…"). Instead of getting caught up in those thoughts, close your eyes and concentrate with your breathing on perceiving yourself from within.

VARIATIONS AND SUGGESTIONS
You can try out differing levels of pressure and tenderness, and you may determine that you have different needs and sensations on different days.

Exercise 37: Breast massage for the content, comfortable woman

Sometimes a woman doesn't just want to spoil herself; she wants to be spoiled. Then she has the massage done by someone else.

GOAL
Giving yourself openly and trustingly into the hands of a pleasure companion, and passively feeling and enjoying the breast massage.

TIME AND EXTERNAL PREPARATIONS
About fifteen minutes per partner.

STEP BY STEP
* Sit down in front of your companion, whose legs are spread and who can be leaning up against something. Let your partner massage your breasts in this position.

* Next, stand up with your arms raised high (if you like, hold on to a door frame). Have your masseuse stand directly behind you and massage your breasts this way.

* Lean forward and let your masseuse lean gently on your back, massaging your breasts this way.

* Lie down on your back on top of your partner, who is also lying on her or his back. (If your partner is a woman, it's usually most

comfortable for your sacrum to be resting on her mons veneris.)
Let your partner massage your breasts. Experiment a little to find a
comfortable position where your masseuse can touch your breasts
without too much effort.

✳ Close by giving your partner a response and a thank-you.

✳ Afterward, you can switch roles.

CREATIVE WAYS TO DEAL WITH STUMBLING BLOCKS
If you're the masseuse, maybe sometimes you don't dare change an uncomfortable position because you don't want to disturb the person being massaged. Again, remember: better a small disruption from a change in position than a large disruption from you transmitting your muscle cramps to your partner.

VARIATIONS AND SUGGESTIONS
If you massage each other regularly, each of you will either develop a preferred method or find that you prefer different methods, depending on the day. Such preferences are best communicated by clearly expressing your wishes in an atmosphere of openness and loving contact.

🦢 Exercise 38: Gladdening the heart in three-part harmony

Most of us are used to sharing the most intimate spaces of our lives with, at most, one person we trust. That's often brave enough. Here we go a step further, with three-way erotic pampering where each person can have the wonderful experience of being spoiled by two stroking organisms. This means no longer registering the individual touches separately, and as a result being able to succumb even more and to revel in your own pleasure. Corresponding to the tantric teaching of the spots where kisses are usually the most effective, here various spots are visited and tenderly spoiled. And through deep breaths on the heart level, each little gratification gladdens the heart as well.

Many women have had painful experiences in which they actually wanted to experience more sensual-erotic pleasures but then felt compelled to have sexual contacts, or at least they placed themselves under that kind of pressure. What I describe below is a very strictly regulated massage that can create a counterbalance to those negative, automatic impulses, as long as all three agree ahead of time that they are meeting to perform this ritual without having any claims on one another later.

GOAL

Gladdening the heart by experiencing tenderness, gentleness, and eroticism without sexuality in the narrower sense and without the expectation that these feelings can be experienced only with a high degree of intimacy between two people.

TIME AND EXTERNAL PREPARATIONS

Three segments of about an hour each, with breaks and time for discussion and conclusion afterward. You may need a blanket. As preparation for a particularly effective massage, it is recommended that you take a few minutes to practice sexual breathing (see Exercise 15), which is felt especially at the heart level, or, if you love one another already, you can indulge in a little round of compliments and caresses.

STEP BY STEP

* *As the enjoyer,* you alone determine the places where you do not want to be touched at all, or not in a certain way; you can, of course, change your mind at any time during the massage and let the others know. The same applies if you would like to receive gentler or firmer touches. The pleasure companions should see themselves as givers and servants of the person being massaged.

* In this erotic massage, various erogenous zones are touched in the following specific order:
  - first very gently with the fingertips
  - then with the breath, blowing hot or cold
  - and finally with the tip of the tongue

* *As the recipient,* begin by lying on your stomach, your forehead supported on your hands. *Pleasure companions,* after briefly consulting and agreeing on how nonsymmetrical zones will be

divided up, begin by touching the following erogenous zones in the three ways described above:

— the recipient's neck area and sacrum

— the knee joints and inner thighs

✳ Now carefully roll the enjoyer over onto her back , and touch the following erogenous zones in all three ways:

— both pinky fingers

— both ears

— lips and navel

— breasts, including the nipples

— pubic bone and inner thighs

— both big toes

✳ Throughout this whole experience, enjoyer, your main job is to use your breath to guide all these pleasant sensations into your heart region, and to take them in like delicious food for the soul. If any unpleasant memories come up, you should halt the memories immediately and breathe out forcefully, imagining that you are passing this experience into the ground or the air.

✳ In order to let all these touches take their effect inside her without distraction, the recipient is left alone for a moment at the end (covered up, if she likes).

✳ When changing roles, a short transitional action is recommended, such as shaking yourselves, drinking water, or changing the music, without too much talking.

✳ The in-depth discussion happens after the exercise has been completed.

CREATIVE WAYS TO DEAL WITH STUMBLING BLOCKS

When partners like each other very much but don't know each other very well yet, there is often resistance to the licking—on the part of the recipient, the companions, or all three. It is important here to set boundaries right away, rather than being disgusted or feeling otherwise uncomfortable.

Instead of licking, you could, for example, use your fingers to drip water from a small bowl onto each spot.

The recipient may not want to be touched in certain places. It is important that her companions truly respect this. If the recipient feels that her boundaries are being acknowledged and respected, she may try expanding them a little herself. (This is completely different from crossing someone else's boundaries!)

🐚 Exercise 39: Kundalini massage

Kundalini energy is *the* sexual force, the one that usually lies sleeping, coiled like a snake at the base of your spine. With the right stimulation it can be set in motion, snaking upward and filling the whole woman with the serpentine movements of its sexual energy.

GOAL
Awakening the power of kundalini and guiding the kundalini energy up through the spine.

TIME AND EXTERNAL PREPARATIONS
Two segments of about an hour each, plus time for discussion afterward. You need a sufficiently large, sensually decorated love nest.

STEP BY STEP
* After a heart-to-heart embrace while standing up (see Exercise 25), both partners relax into the nicely decorated love nest, and the pleasure companion slowly and carefully undresses the recipient, possibly adding a few honest compliments.

* Kundalini breathing: In this breathing exercise, which the recipient will continue throughout the whole massage, the concentration is on the spine. *If you are the recipient,* as you breathe in through your mouth, move your rump slightly backward, and then let a wave move upward through your whole body as you exhale. This wave is not an exertion, but rather something you let happen.

* Beginning of the kundalini massage: The recipient, naked, lies on her belly and begins to practice kundalini breathing.

✳ *If you are the pleasure companion,* establish contact with the recipient's spine by laying your hand on the recipient's sacrum and breathing along with the recipient.

✳ Then use your fingertips to tap lightly, bending from the wrist, all over the whole sacrum, like a gentle rain. Here, as in the rest of the massage, it is important that you be sitting comfortably, so that you transmit only pleasurable energy and not tension.

✳ Next, cross your thumbs and massage the recipient, using only your thumbs. Use strong pressure to stroke the right and left sides of the spine, from the sacrum to the base of the skull.

✳ After that, draw the flat of your hand along the left side of the spine up to your partner's neck; massage the neck in short clockwise circles, and then return along the right side of the spine.

✳ Then the main part of the massage begins: Find the kundalini point at the end of the coccyx or tailbone (at the top of the cleft of the buttocks). It sometimes can be felt as somewhat spongy tissue at the end of the bone. For the recipient, the kundalini point feels either hot, vibrating, or ringing from the inside.

✳ Once you have found the kundalini point (for right-handed people, the right index or middle finger is usually best), quickly vibrate it. (A cellist would say, "Like the vibrato on the high A string.") The vibration should not be directed downward, but rather toward the skull, that is, through the spine. When you have vibrated like this for a while, begin to use the thumb and index finger of your other hand to vibrate your way up, inch by inch, along the discs and vertebrae toward your partner's head. Do this as a question-and-answer exercise: First your right hand vibrates the kundalini point, then your left hand vibrates the lowermost part of the sacrum. The right hand vibrates the kundalini point again, while the left hand moves up a tiny bit toward the head and vibrates as if responding to the other hand.

✳ While the two hands are still relatively close together, the question-and-answer can be faster; the greater the distance between the two, the more time it may take to give an "answer."

✳ When you reach the back side of the heart, advance more slowly with your left hand so that the heart region is very clearly connected with the sexual force.

✳ When you reach the nape of your partner's neck, ask your partner to support her forehead with both hands so that her neck is not bent.

✳ Then, when you reach the base of the skull, vibrate not just in the middle, but all the way out to the ears and back before moving up along the back of the head to the crown, using extremely gentle vibrations.

✳ Finish off the contact by synchronously vibrating your fingers at the coccyx and the crown. After a short time, carefully release your fingers, and squat at the level of your partner's sacrum.

✳ Make sure your lips are dry, and brush them across the top of the cleft of the buttocks without touching it (at a distance of about half an inch), while blowing warm or even hot air toward the kundalini point. Treat the whole spine to this breath, moving upward inch by inch until you have reached the nape of your partner's neck. Again, linger attentively in the heart region.

✳ You can also simply blow up and down the spine a few more times, but sometimes this feels too cold on the recipient's warmed-up back; in addition, the hot air from the depth of your body brings more flow.

✳ When you have reached the top, you can also give the recipient several hot, dry, feather-light kisses at the nape of the neck (which is also an orgasmic point).

✳ At the end, lay one hand on the coccyx and one on the nape of the neck or base of the skull, breathe deeply and regularly, and pour calmness through your hands into the recipient's body.

* Then slowly release your hands; do not touch the recipient anymore, but remain near her and inwardly connected with her, so that she can sense the energy without having to direct her attention to the room or other external conditions.

* If you lie or sit next to each other for a while to discuss the experience before switching roles, the first recipient determines your position, proximity, and the nature of your talking or silence.

CREATIVE WAYS TO DEAL WITH STUMBLING BLOCKS

Since this massage will be unfamiliar to most people, they often need to begin by working on the strength and direction of the vibration until it feels right and is at a tempo where the recipient can really feel the flow of energy. It is important that the recipient not criticize the companion harshly. Instead, use your hand to demonstrate what you would like. Also, both of you should experiment until what you are doing feels good to both of you.

Women with large breasts sometimes find lying on their stomachs more comfortable if they place a pillow under their breasts.

Sometimes it's also nice to have a pillow under your ankles, because it takes the pressure off your joints and foot bones.

VARIATIONS AND SUGGESTIONS

Some recipients like to be helped to their feet after a short period of meditation, so that they can feel their kundalini energy develop upward with a subtly rising vibration.

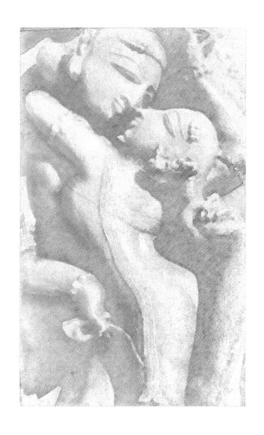

☙ CHAPTER 8 ❧

Rituals of
Transformation

*U*nlike other cultures, we are short on rituals dealing with things like transitions between phases of development or creating new identities. Rituals of Western culture tend to focus on performing and functioning. For example, we lack a ritual to celebrate a girl's first period as the symbol of becoming a woman or to recognize menopause as a transition into the identity of a wise woman. Spiritual movements and even tantric groups try to make up for this lack by translating rituals from other times and cultures, and reshaping them for our needs. I myself have not adopted any rituals the way I learned them, but have tried to develop them further, according to my interests and those of the women in my groups.

Overall, for sexual rituals, even more so than for rituals focusing on other aspects of life, the following words ring true:

Even eternity is made up of moments,

And every intensely enjoyed moment is a pearl of love on the string
of your lifetime.

Time is the soul of the world.

It is up to us to ignore it or smile upon it.

So experience every second of your being with all your senses, and stretch your time out more and more in the direction of intensely experienced slowness.

On the Structure of Rituals

Particularly for rituals dealing with sensuality, eroticism, and sexuality, it is important to create a protected space where each individual can feel safe and strengthened. Beyond that, the following general steps should be taken when executing spiritual rituals:

* Draw a protective circle around yourselves (e.g., with a stick or a piece of incense) so that you can feel undisturbed and protected in your nest.

* Strive for inner purification, so that there are as few sensitivity-hindering shadows and waste materials as possible in your body of

energy (your aura). When you feel a great deal of stress in yourselves or in the room, for example, wave a glowing sage bushel
around, then air out the room. For getting rid of waste matter,
for example lactic acid buildup in tense muscles, shake yourself
or dance wildly. For a more subtle cleansing of your body of
energy, use your hand to waft the golden or white pomander from
the Aura-Soma collection into your aura (ask for it in spiritual
bookshops or go to www.aura-soma.net). For confusion and
strong outward orientation, sprinkle salt water on the chakra of
the third eye.

✳ Call on the four elements. You may also call upon the power of the
deep (e.g., the survival strength of your generous grandmother), of
the heights (e.g., your inspirations from dreams and visions), and
of the middle (e.g., the power of self-healing that each of us
possesses) in order to make these forces conscious in the forming
of each participant, and to activate them.

✳ Call on Tara or other goddesses, and possibly on female friends or
ancestors, who will accompany and promote the ritual so that you
can feel supported and receive spiritual help in difficult phases.

✳ Tune in to one another so that you can relate to each other clearly.

✳ Formulate wishes, goals, and boundaries.

✳ Complete each ritual.

✳ Take leave of the goddess(es) and powers with a word of thanks or
a word about their effects on you, which will not disappear even if
your attention is now directed elsewhere.

✳ Honor the place, for example by leaving a flower as a symbol of
the powers of transformation or, if you're indoors, by physically
cleaning and returning the room to its previous state.

✳ Remove the circle.

(For more information about these aspects of ritual, read, for example,
Rituals of Healing: Using Imagery for Health and Wellness, by Jeanne
Achterberg. See "Inspirational Literature" in the Resources section.)

SUGGESTION FOR CALLING THE FOUR ELEMENTS

The four elements—water, fire, earth, air—as bearers of our lives are naturally present in every process, every person, and every group. Nevertheless, it helps to have symbolic objects and verbal supplications at the ready to activate the characteristics of each element in every participant, and to make her aware of how she is living out and enlivening the qualities of these elements in her life at the present time.

The elements connected with spiritual and emotional principles are similar in many cultures, but the compass points, for example, to which they are assigned can be very different. My connections follow the medicine wheel of the Cherokees, but if participants prefer to make other connections, they are certainly welcome to do so.

SUGGESTIONS FOR SYMBOLIC OBJECTS

Water: a jug containing tap water or salt water

Fire: a burning candle, lamp, glowing coal, or incense stick

Earth: a handful of earth in a bowl, a stone, potted plant, clay pot, pentagram, or carved figure (one that embodies solidity, security, or nourishing qualities)

Air: bird feathers, a fan, pinwheel, balloon, or sword (tarot)

SUGGESTIONS FOR SUPPLICATIONS

At the beginning of each supplication, one of you takes a symbolic object, goes to the corresponding compass point outside the circle, and turns her face in this direction.

Water: "I call upon the goddess (the power) of the East, the blue spirit of water and flowing energy, the principle of softness in love that flows throughout the whole living world. Help us to give and to receive; help us to feel the ebb and flow within us and in nature around us; help us to give in to the tides within us."

Fire: "I call upon the goddess (the power) of the South, the red spirit of fire and passion, of blood, sexuality, and vital warmth, the driving forces of striving, the power and joy of ecstasy. Help us to express our emotions creatively for ourselves and for others.

Help us to live fully and completely. Warm our hearts and our fiery places."

Earth: "I call upon the goddess (the power) of the West, the golden spirit of the earth and of creation, the principle of fruitfulness, the strength of regeneration and renewal. Help us to settle in the lap of Mother Earth, to heal her wounds and to live together in peace as her children. Help us to understand the processes of living and dying, when to sow and when to reap."

Air: "I call upon the goddess (the power) of the North, the white spirit of winter, of death and even the small death of love, the consideration of what is important in our lives, the wise and timeless old woman who knows the secrets of eternity. Help us to breathe unhindered, to drink the winds and to find our quiet center. Help us to develop a free spirit and to recognize, with crystal clarity, what we need to know. Help us to think quickly and to see without distortion."

These supplications can be elaborated with the powers of earth and heaven (below and above) and with your ancestors or other helpful connecting beings.

This is followed by a supplication to the middle, for example with objects symbolizing Tara (like a picture or a small statue), which can give the individual participant strength.

For undesirable beings, a bowl of rice can be set outside the circle, with instructions telling them to enjoy themselves and then leave in peace.

SUGGESTIONS FOR TAKING LEAVE OF THE POWERS AND GODDESSES AFTER THE RITUAL

1. Those participants who have called on the powers/elements should face the corresponding compass points once more at the end, thank these powers, and say good-bye to them. The other person (or other people) looks in the same direction.

2. Next, perform a quick reclaiming of the powers (as explained by ritual guide Maria Zemp):

Earth: shuffle your feet

Air: click your tongue

Fire: clap your hands

Water: click with your tongue against the roof of your mouth

These sounds symbolically release the powers of each element back to their respective compass points, recognizing their effects once more without requiring too many words at the end of the ritual.

3. After that, you can use the following chant to reopen the circle:

By the earth, which is our pleasure-ready body,

by the air, which is our deep breath,

by the fire, which fans our sexual heat,

and by the waters of our living lap,

by our ancestresses below us,

by our visions above us,

and by the middle of our feeling heart,

there, where our inner Tara rests—

the circle is now open, yet unbroken.

We found our way to each other,

now we go our own ways—

and maybe we will meet again.

⚐ Exercise 40: Ritual to awaken the senses

Like the elements, our senses are always present, drawing the powers of the outside world into us and directing them within us. And just as our body is the space for our sexuality, our senses are the openings through which pleasures enter that room and set the body vibrating.

In our everyday lives, we are forced to close these openings fairly often so that we aren't overwhelmed by an excess of stimuli, coming in a too-rapid and chaotic succession. This creates a deficiency of stimuli within us and a longing for intensity. In this ritual, the hunger for intensity is satisfied with a few concentrated, slowly and carefully offered stimuli, which have a far greater effect than large amounts of replacement objects (e.g., eating giant servings of spaghetti with the thought, "Noodles make you happy—even more noodles make you even happier!") or relationship dramas (as in, "I fight, therefore I am!").

Experiencing this "spoiling of the senses" creates a feeling of "sense fulfillment," of meaningful existence. And since our society has developed an overemphasis on the visual senses, making many people glad when they have a chance to close their eyes, this ritual instead emphasizes the other senses—in order to awaken them, to improve them, and to make you conscious of their special contributions to pleasurable sexuality.

GOAL

Awakening all the senses (except the sense of seeing, which is activated only at the end) and encouraging you to give in to the unknown.

TIME AND EXTERNAL PREPARATIONS

About an hour.

Preparations for the pleasure companion

Preheat the room; cut fruit into small pieces and arrange them with nuts and chocolates; prepare drinks and water glasses; have recorded music or instruments ready along with feathers and scented oils.

Preparations for the enjoyer

Make yourself pretty and scantily clad (more skin showing means more pleasure…). Prepare a welcoming gift (e.g., a small flower arrangement, a beautiful stone, a scented oil) that you will hand over to your companion when you receive her.

If the musical accompaniment for each phase of the ritual is to be more than just background music—instead, an exquisite encouragement for each of the senses—a CD or tape recording custom-made with appropriate pieces is recommended. For examples, see the following table:

✳ MUSIC FOR THE RITUAL TO AWAKEN THE SENSES

Steps	Music
1. leading to the spot, blindfolded	*Adagio* (from nearly any classical music sampler)
2. tuning in to the heart	complete silence!
3. singing the Tara mantra	no music in the background
4. musical instruments	no music in the background
5. scented oils	*Lands of the Dawn* (tracks 2, 3, 5)
6. water	*Mega Sound Effects Vol. 2* (tracks 1, 6)
7. fanning the wind	*Mega Sound Effects Vol. 2* (track 12)
8. feeding with fruits	*Like an Endless River* (track 3)
9. feathers	*Like an Endless River* (track 6)
10. leaning/protecting	*Like an Endless River* (track 5)
11. waltz	Viennese waltz (sampler)
12. removing blindfold	continuation of the waltz
13. leading back to the bed	*Garten der Liebe* (*Garden of Love*; track 2)
14. discussion with each other	*Listening to the Heart* (track 3, 6)

(Further information on the music listed above is given in the Resources section.)

STEP BY STEP

Setting the mood (recipient)

* *You, the recipient:* For once, allow yourself to open up with all your senses (except for the often-dominant sense of sight)…to broaden, to open yourself with every single pore…to open yourself fully and completely…not just to the unknown experiences that await you…not just to your fairy or pleasure companion… but above all to your own primeval sensuality!

* Prepare your senses to receive!

* Trust in your fairy's desire to spoil you deliciously—she will do so!

✳ Let yourself become still and open and curious—especially about yourself and your sensations!

✳ Become an unconcerned child who wants to explore the world of the senses; a mature, red-blooded adult who wants to drink life to the fullest; a wise elder who loves life in its simplicity and who quietly, contentedly enjoys it—all at once.

✳ Nothing is important right now besides enjoying the moment!

✳ And if you feel a pleasurable sensation, take a deep breath and pull it upward to your heart! There you can take it in as food for the soul, which your heart will transform into the subtle energy of love. You can experience this as openness, devotion, and receptiveness, as gentle movements within you, as goodness and expansiveness.

✳ If different thoughts disturb you, don't give them any more energy; don't fight with them, but let them flow out of you with your next exhalation, and fill yourself with new life energy as you breathe in.

✳ In a loving way, say if you don't like something or if you need something (a pillow, for example)—your fairy will do everything in her power for you.

✳ Now is the time to devote yourself, with dignity, to your senses, to your feelings, to yourself!

✳ When, in a moment, you knock on the door, blindfolded, pause in the door frame and ask loudly, "Where is the magic fairy who will lead me into the realm of the senses?"

Setting the mood (pleasure companion)

✳ *You, the pleasure companion:* Become a magic fairy today, one who might learn a new way to enchant and to serve.

✳ Yes, serving is a job with which we women have been burdened for centuries. Let us be glad that we, as feminists, are able to develop clearly recognizable resistances here and want to neither rule nor serve in our regular lives.

* In the tantric spoiling ritual, imagine a kind of serving where you maintain your dignity as a woman and at the same time devote yourself completely to making another person feel good. That means tuning in all your activities, your ideas, and even your ways of walking and breathing to the recipient.

* You are testing out the silent joy of devoting yourself to the recipient's pleasure. Nothing else is important now besides *her* maximal pleasure through you.

* This becomes possible when you connect your heart to hers, letting every hand movement come from the movements of your heart, and then enchant her with an attentive heart...enchant her into a realm of simplicity, simple sensuality, and tender silence.

* Of course you have a couple of magic tricks up your sleeve, but those are just aids for the tender magic strength of your devotion to *her* pleasure! Spoil her with the placid twinkle of a magic fairy who knows how much power lies in her devotion to the other's pleasure and how much joy lies in fusing with something beyond her own wishes and needs.

* When, in a moment, your pleasure recipient knocks on the door and asks you a question, you will take her hand and lead her to your decorated love nest. There you will make sure she is sitting comfortably. Remind yourself of how sensitive she is when she cannot see anything and is trusting you blindly.

For the ritual together

* The pleasure companion sits across from the recipient and inwardly tunes in to her; in the same way, the recipient inwardly tunes in to the companion. Both animate the recipient's heart chakra with deep, gentle breaths. And above all, the companion knows that all stimuli are really just the outer paths to a heart-to-heart encounter. In order to tune in to each other even more on a mental level, the recipient can, for example, think about the Tara quality of patience and devotion, while the companion considers the Tara quality of generosity. Both the companion and the recipi-

ent, by singing the Tara mantra together (see Chapter I), call these qualities into being in themselves and bind them to one another, just as these qualities are bound together in Tara.

✳ Companion, reach for a musical instrument and quietly make a sound with it in order to gladden the recipient's ears as you walk around her. (The instruments can be changed a few times, or the companion could instead sing or hum.)

✳ Hold various scented oils under the recipient's nose, waving the scent toward her and playing with it a little in front of her nostrils.

✳ After playing water music (for example, ocean or river music), sprinkle the recipient's bare skin with water from a cold bowl. Off and on, tease or give pleasant shivers to the recipient with the cold mist from a spray bottle.

✳ Take the bowl containing pieces of fruit, nuts, and chocolates, and slowly feed the recipient, letting her smell the food first and touching her lips to it. During this exercise, some companions turn into mischievous witches, only letting their partner briefly smell the truffle, then warming it up on her nipples and drawing on her breasts and clavicle with it and teasing her lips with the rest....

✳ After eating there is wind music, and accordingly the recipient is fanned with fans or cloths. This can be a warm summer wind or even a hefty autumn storm from the repertoire of a not-always-gentle magic fairy.

✳ Begin to touch and stroke all the bared skin of the recipient with one or two large feathers, first moving only in the recipient's aura and then directly touching the skin.

✳ Smoothe out the recipient's aura. Do this by stroking with your hands one-half to one inch above the skin, where you can feel an invisible "skin" because of the warmth or a subtle tingling in your palms, as though you were smoothing out a silk cloth. Now help the recipient to her feet. Give the recipient a heart-to-heart embrace (see Exercise 25) and remain standing with her until you have the impression that she is steady on her feet again.

✳ With Viennese waltz music (if space is limited or you are out of practice, a slow waltz or anything swinging will do), lead the recipient into the dance.

✳ After the first waltz, remove the blindfold; the next waltz is danced with open eyes.

✳ Both of you return to your nest and, accompanied by quiet music, discuss your feelings and experiences. Look again at the gift accepted by the companion at the beginning of the ritual. You can lie next to each other for a while and let the ritual come to an end.

CREATIVE WAYS TO DEAL WITH STUMBLING BLOCKS
Some recipients do not deal well with the tension of not knowing, and they begin to talk or move uneasily. If you notice yourself doing this, breathe deeply and think about pleasurable anticipation.

Some people find long periods of sitting uncomfortable, or they get cold easily. Let your companion know if this happens, and she will quickly come to your aid.

VARIATIONS AND SUGGESTIONS
You can, of course, also switch roles during this ritual. However, sometimes it's a more lasting experience if you remain in one role and play it out completely. You can take on the other role the next time.

🍃 Exercise 41: Rose ritual

In early summer, when the first roses bloom, you can also encourage the blooming of tender feelings in your heart through sensual experiences with this flower of love. The rose ritual improves your devotions to your own tenderness.

GOAL
Pampering your partner with rose petals, rose scents, and pictures of roses in order to emphasize the tender aspects of her capacity to love.

TIME AND EXTERNAL PREPARATIONS
About an hour per partner, plus time for an exchange afterward. In addition:

✳ Prepare two bowls, each containing the petals from at least twenty to thirty roses and a rose blossom without stem or leaves.

✳ Prepare rose water by adding a few drops of rose oil to water in a spray bottle.

✳ Prepare a rose scent in an oil burner (Mexican or Moroccan rose is best, since they are less sweet and cloying than tea rose), or light a stick of rose-scented incense.

✳ Set aside two rose quartzes.

✳ Prepare a sensual love nest on a large mat, decorated with beautiful cloths and maybe surrounded by flowers and ritual objects.

STEP BY STEP

✳ The two partners sit facing each other, very close but without actually touching.

✳ Both of you close your eyes, lay a hand on your own heart, and breathe deeply and regularly, emphasizing chest breathing. Each of you concentrate on your heart and on the sensations you detect in your heart chakra at this moment.

✳ Now each of you imagine that your heart chakra is growing larger and larger with each breath. This is not physical growth, but rather the spread of heart energy within the body. As this area spreads out more and more, you can imagine that a rosebud is slowly growing in your heart region. The rose opens a little more with each breath, letting its beauty bloom forth, and begins to spread its scent through the body. This scent finally flows out beyond the borders of your body and fills the room with the subtle scent of the flower of love.

✳ Then each of you take your free hand and find your partner's heart hand, laying your hand on top of your partner's. A bond between the roses and the heart energies is created by the flow through your arms and hands.

✳ Remain connected with your partner for a while through imagination and touch. Imagine that the scents of your two roses are commingling. You may also imagine that your combined scent is filling the room, working as an atmospheric protection against any intruders and continually reaffirming your bond with each other.

✳ Now remove your hands from the other's chakra, then your hands from your own hearts. Meditate for a moment and then open your eyes. Look at each other with the wide gaze of an open heart, and allow the other to look into your eyes, seeing all the way to your heart.

✳ Then each of you take one of the little bowls with the rose petals and the one rose blossom. Pick up the rose, and take turns pulling off petals and laying them in the other's bowl, along with an honest, heartfelt compliment. This can last as long as there are petals remaining but can also be cut shorter. If you run out of ideas for compliments, you can always repeat and reinforce things that have already been said.

✳ Now agree upon your roles as enjoyer and pleasure companion, which will be reversed at the end.

✳ *If you're the pleasure companion,* carefully undress the enjoyer and place her clothes to the side. Help the enjoyer to lie down comfortably on her back. The enjoyer is allowed to express any last wishes before silently giving in to the subtle pleasures that await. Now slowly and carefully begin to place single rose petals on the recipient's body. You can, for example, decorate the recipient with single petals in sensitive areas; you can form little piles of petals on her body; you can gently use petals to stroke under the recipient's fingertips, making her aware of the petals' velvety properties; you can blow little clusters of petals across the recipient's body; you can cover the body's openings, folds, and furrows with rose petals, growing more and more unselfconsciously involved in the game yourself.

✳ Accompanied now by energetic music (a pop song involving roses, perhaps), you can reach a crescendo by letting more rose petals fall onto the recipient from a greater height, massaging her with the petals, drawing large circles on her, and energetically covering as many of her body parts as possible with rose petals before blowing the petals in all directions.

✳ Now give the recipient another chance to express any fantasies or wishes, ways she would like to be touched or covered with rose petals, or be bedded upon them. You can hold an intense rose scent under the recipient's nose in the form of a scented oil, and finally spray any skin not covered in petals with rose-scented water.

✳ The whole time, enjoyer, remember that if a touch or other sensation feels good, take it into your heart with a deep breath and keep it there forever. And if a touch feels unfamiliar or strange, breathe even more deeply in order to see whether or not it feels good. And if something doesn't feel good, release the feeling with a powerful exhalation. Then give your companion the chance to spoil you even more by telling her, in a brief and friendly manner, what you don't want or what you would rather have done differently. You can be sure that a companion who is tuned in to your heart will do *everything* to make the experience better for you!

✳ At the end, the companion lays a rose quartz on the recipient's heart chakra, covers her up if she likes, and leaves her alone for a little while (without touching her, but also without physically leaving her) so that she can meditate on the various rose-petal touches she has experienced.

✳ Now take a short break to rearrange the love nest, get a drink, or go to the bathroom, but without talking too much.

✳ After you have exchanged roles and performed the second rose ritual, you can lie beside each other for a while, enjoy a phase of mutual silence, and then discuss what you have experienced.

CREATIVE WAYS TO DEAL WITH STUMBLING BLOCKS
Some pleasure companions are afraid they will not think of enough things to do with the petals. It helps to imagine playing like a young child in a summer meadow and to just leave it up to your hands and the specific properties of the rose petals to please your recipient.

During the course of the ritual, some recipients feel resistance to opening themselves up further and criticize themselves for it. If you notice this happening, allow yourself a moment to recognize and express your sorrow or anger at "not yet being able to open up all the way," and then concentrate on the kind of opening up that is possible for you right now.

VARIATIONS AND SUGGESTIONS

This ritual can have an even stronger effect if it can be done outside in a sunny summer meadow where there is a gentle breeze, birds are chirping, and no human or animal disruption is likely.

🌀 Exercise 42: Women's demonstration of two yonis

This women's demonstration is an expedition into sexual worlds of symbols, and it helps you come to terms with your extrapersonal qualities.

GOAL

By seeing others and having your own yoni be seen in its extrapersonal qualities, you can develop a deeper understanding of your own female identity.

TIME AND EXTERNAL PREPARATIONS

About thirty to forty minutes for the demonstration, then time for discussion. Clothing: A simple sarong is best; that is, a cloth slung around your hips, beneath which you are naked. The clothing lends itself to a room that is nice and warm. Background music with a very light rhythm can help "carry" you.

STEP BY STEP

* After a slow heart-to-heart embrace (see Exercise 25), the two partners sit across from each other with closed sarongs, without touching.

* First agree on the order in which you will take the roles of "displayer" and "gazer."

* *If you are the displayer,* open your sarong and show the gazer your

yoni, in such a way that you are sitting comfortably while still affording your partner a good view.

✳ *If you are the gazer,* look with the soft gaze of an open heart, but also very carefully. Describe what you see with sensual, flowery words, and make honestly meant compliments. The displayer draws each compliment into her yoni and her heart like fluid nourishment, and under no circumstances contradicts the gazer.

✳ Now the gazer imagines the displayer's yoni to be a symbol of every existing yoni, as the Tara yoni or as the sacred lap of Mother Earth. Bow before it as before a temple of pleasure. Here you can experience the connection between sexual glances and spiritually broad gazing.

✳ During this time, the displayer can identify herself with this extrapersonal quality (beyond her personal character) and share the following phrase with the gazer: "I am your beginning, and I am your end."

✳ Now, gazer, imagine that the yoni you see before you is the lap of your own mother, out of which you slipped many years ago. Express your feelings and associations about this.

✳ Displayer, since you know that your partner is not referring personally to you here, allow yourself to take in all these words calmly without relating them back to yourself.

✳ Gazer, imagine that this yoni is the yoni of a woman who once hurt or left you. Investigate whether you have forgiven your former lover or can forgive her now. Say so only if it is honestly possible. Otherwise, express any feelings that come up.

✳ Displayer, do not take these words personally either. Instead, concentrate on the sensations of well-being you can now feel in your yoni. End the sequence by saying, "The pleasure and power of my yoni are indestructible," and cover yourself again.

✳ After an appropriate pause, switch roles.

∗ Before you discuss your experiences, each of you lie down or sit peacefully for a moment and meditate on your own sensations.

CREATIVE WAYS TO DEAL WITH STUMBLING BLOCKS
In order to avoid growing emotional, one or both partners may start talking. Save the talk for later so that you don't talk the tender shoots of feelings into the ground.

Some people have trouble with this type of ceremoniousness and find themselves laughing. Allow yourself to breathe deeply, to be deeply touched, and to express what is going on in your innermost being.

VARIATIONS AND SUGGESTIONS
If one of you is particularly close to a goddess or to a real woman, or is particularly conflicted about someone, you can experiment with your image of that woman's yoni. If your feelings grow too strong and you no longer feel secure in the encounter, you can break it off at any time and calmly explain it to your partner as needed. In this situation, an especially loving mutual conclusion to the demonstration is necessary.

🍃 Exercise 43: Self-love ritual in the presence of another

The enjoyment of sexual self-love alone in your quiet little room—in a society like ours with so much disrespect for women and the lack of self-respect that results from it—cannot be taken for granted. Self-love in the consciously chosen presence of another person requires even more courage to show yourself vulnerably, ecstatically, and very intimately. That's why this is a more advanced exercise.

GOAL
Opening up your own intimacy boundaries for another person of your choosing, and the brave and proud display of yourself experiencing your own pleasure.

TIME AND EXTERNAL PREPARATIONS
At least an hour for each partner, plus discussion time afterward. You need a comfortable and serviceable love nest with beautiful cloths, powerful objects, beverages, and love tools within reach.

STEP BY STEP

✳ The self-lover and her passive companion, sitting, first tune in to each other with their breathing and their loving attention to each other. The self-lover decides where the companion/observer will sit and whether the companion can help if needed (passing the massage oil, etc.) or should stay passive on the periphery.

✳ If possible, the companion/observer breathes in rhythm with the self-lover, focusing the eyes less on exact concentration and more on a broad, warm gaze from the heart, one that can take in the atmosphere and permit emotions to arise.

✳ *If you're the self-lover,* with your eyes closed, now concentrate on yourself in the presence of another. Remind yourself that *you* are the most important person in the process of self-love, and that you will not let yourself be disturbed by any power in the world.

✳ You can also call on helpful spirits (e.g., your scrappy grandma's sense of humor or the goddess Tara) and ban unloving spirits (e.g., a strictly controlling mother) from your surroundings (see "Cleaning out your overflowing love nest," Exercise 23).

✳ Now begin to undress yourself slowly and mindfully, gradually beginning to touch your hands and arms, and then touching, exploring, teasing, stroking, and caressing every part of your body as though it were the body of an unknown lover.

✳ Every so often you can open your eyes and see yourself in the other's gaze, and in moments of uncertainty or self-criticism, you can breathe in the (hopefully) loving, joyful gaze of your partner.

✳ Occasionally, the companion can give the self-lover a compliment on her body or on her way of loving herself (provided, of course, that they have not agreed to remain completely silent). Here, as at other times, compliments are only effective when they are honest and come from the heart.

✳ Then, self-lover, fan the flames of your sexual fire higher and higher by focusing your activities on your favorite erogenous zones: lips, earlobes, nipples, loins, inner thighs, knees, mons veneris, labia, clitoris, vagina, perineum....

* Every so often, look into the eyes of your companion and seek the mirror of your own pleasure in them.

* Observer, even if you get so aroused that you'd like to "lend a hand," refrain from doing so; instead, breathe the arousal deep into your heart and, at most, use it to give a compliment to your partner.

* In this love game with yourself, it is less important whether you reach orgasmic ecstasy or other high levels of arousal, than whether you stick with forms of tenderness and affection for yourself. What is important is your loving relationship with yourself and your attempt to show yourself to another person, courageously and with an awareness of your own dignity.

* Self-lover, after you have experienced your own kind of climax or high point, slowly bring the stimulating movements to an end, allowing yourself to pay attention to the overtones until you finally come to rest and are given a moment to yourself.

* Then you can order your companion to sit or lie down next to you, hold your hand or your head, and talk with you a little about both of your experiences.

* After that, switch roles, and then spend a longer time discussing the experience.

CREATIVE WAYS TO DEAL WITH STUMBLING BLOCKS
Some women place enormous pressure on themselves to have an orgasm because of the other person's presence. This usually guarantees that orgasmic high points will remain out of reach. Also, some women do not experience orgasms in the conventional sense of the word and will criticize themselves because of it. In both cases, remember: It isn't about the short phase of one or more climaxes; it's about the phase of being tender with yourself, of self-arousal, of the flow and the shape of self-love, however this might be possible (with the hindrances that still exist) for you at the moment.

VARIATIONS AND SUGGESTIONS

Here's a more advanced variation: Self-lover, before gliding into the act of self-love, concentrate on what your mother would say right now. Share this statement with your companion, who remembers it. In a phase of great arousal, suddenly imagine that your companion is transformed into your mother, who says the statement to you. The companion does so when you ask her, and you allow yourself to feel the effects of the words spoken. Then imagine how you might respond to this motherly phrase with all your pride as an adult. For example: "There, Mother, now you see all the things a woman like me can do!" or, "Go ahead and watch for a minute, Mother, because you can learn a few things from me!"

✒ Exercise 44: Queen game

What do medieval minority occupations have to do with the age of feminism? Well, just as we sometimes have to "borrow" from other cultures because our own is impoverished, we can also "borrow" from other eras in order to pick out a skill we can use today (without necessarily idealizing all other times or cultures in general, or copying them completely). For with all our attempts to fight for equal rights for women on a societal level, we sometimes overemphasize our sameness rather than enjoying the benefits of *temporary inequality*.

GOAL

Learning two important roles for developing sexual creativity: smart ruling and conscious serving from the heart. Learning one role promotes training in the other.

TIME AND EXTERNAL PREPARATIONS

Preferably three to five hours for each partner, with a long break (possibly even a whole day) in between. Have handy pens and paper for writing down wishes, and everything you might need for a pleasant love nest. In addition, prepare various music, snacks, and drinks.

STEP BY STEP

    ✳ First, each of you sit down away from the other and think about
       your greatest sexual wishes, your taboos, your boundaries, and the

practicality of various longings. Then place yourself in the role of a powerful but kind queen who would like to be spoiled for hours on end. Bravely write down all the wishes that go along with your imagined scenario and put them in a (tentative) order.

✳ When both of you are finished, decide who will be queen first and when the first phase should start.

✳ Internally prepare for your roles, and dress yourselves according to your perceptions of the role.

✳ *Queen,* you are a very smart ruler. You know what you want, are honest with yourself and the other person, are open to new suggestions, and require of your servant only what she can realistically do power-wise, technically/organizationally, acrobatically, and according to her personality. On the other hand, you order your servant to perform acts of maximum servitude so that you can be sexually spoiled to the greatest extent possible. And here's the most important thing: You become an artist at switching between expressing desires, making corrections, etc., and absolute submission to the moment.

✳ *Servant,* you do not play a victim's role (medieval or modern); you retain your pride while doing everything you can to spoil your mistress as much as possible. This only works if you open your heart so wide that you can include the other person. Any ideas that come to you about your own upcoming role as queen are shelved for now. Put all your creativity, all your playfulness into the practice of your role as an excellent servant of pleasure.

✳ Either of you can say "Stop!" or another agreed-upon code word to immediately end the role-play if you feel uncomfortable or see your dignity being endangered.

✳ Continuously exchange your thoughts on your experiences, yet do so without leaving your roles. You speak *in* your roles but can exaggerate and satirize them. (For example, "O worthy queen, your loving servant is inconsolable that she cannot simultaneously scratch your head, polish your shining red pearl, and hunt with her hands in your royal Venus-forest. My suggestion would be to temporarily withdraw from the Venus-forest, to play in your red-gold hair, and to use this opportunity to tease your Majesty's lips with my tongue. Might this please you?")

* During the game, new ideas may come to you, some of which can be taken up and put into practice in the time remaining. Others can serve as a starting point for future games, for there are limits to the servant's energy and the queen's receptivity.

* At the end, the queen thanks the servant and praises her for the special services rendered. Now leave your roles without immediately slipping into the next ones. A long break—possibly a day—is recommended before switching roles again.

* A lengthy exchange about the experience is sure to be fascinating.

CREATIVE WAYS TO DEAL WITH STUMBLING BLOCKS
If one of you feels overextended or otherwise unwell, you can say "Stop!" at any time and temporarily leave your role in order to think about creatively solving the problem. Then you both resume your roles and stage a second attempt.

If one of you slips out of your role but doesn't say "Stop!" the other emphasizes her own role (rather than leaving it) until the first finds her way back into the game.

VARIATIONS AND SUGGESTIONS
This role play is sometimes even more effective if it's staged in places other than your familiar home, e.g., in nature (as long as it's a place that's both isolated *and* safe), near a swimming pool or hot tub in the midnight hour, in a luxurious hotel room rented for a special rendezvous with your beloved, or wherever else your mutual creativity might open doors....

✐ Exercise 45: Lesbian celebration

Even though in many places the possibility has now opened up for two women to have a "partnership" that is officially recognized in the eyes of the law, this achievement still creates ambivalence in members of various lesbian circles—not just in the sense of rights and justice, but also from the perspective of political strategies; particularly, though, in the sense of the societal formalization of freely chosen love. More and more female couples, however, especially those in long-term relationships, long for acknowledgment and a ceremonial honoring of their love in a larger collective context—and make it sensual, if you please.

Here, then, are a few suggestions for a collective "initiation" into the state of established adult female love, a mutual celebration where guests who have not been tantrically "schooled" but who care about the couple can also take part and celebrate with them.

GOAL
Collective recognition and celebration of a lesbian couple courageous enough to brave marriage.

TIME AND EXTERNAL PREPARATIONS
At least a day; preferably two days. Ask close friends or relatives to help out as organizers. They will plan many of the steps with the two of you but will then take care of the details by themselves. Helpers' assignments might include selecting and practicing music, shopping and preparing food, decorating the rooms or outdoor space, shopping for all the things that are needed. A really fun role is that of ritual mistress, who has the whole thing "under control."

STEP BY STEP

1. Inner and outer cleansing of the two women with each other
The following are some ideas that might require a little preliminary experimentation:

* Individually or with your "intended": Showering, bathing with sensual bath oils, watsu (water shiatsu in a warm swimming pool), rubbing lotion or oil on each other, shaking, and/or sweating (in a sauna or with all the interested parties together in a sweat lodge).

* Enacting a symbolic release from old romantic relationships that could stand in the way of the celebration with the beloved. This happens first through a symbolic binding with the old relationships. Do this by tying each partner with a piece of wool

yarn to people who can stand for the old relationships. Then the current state of closeness to or distance from that person is named; the woman makes an expression of "leftovers" or thanks; and she takes leave of these individuals and/or this type of relationship or encounter, for which there is no room in her new love. She cuts the string as a symbol of separation. Finally, a new coming together of the couple is enacted.

* Saying farewell to any antilesbian norms of the parents or other people close to the couple, to old relationship norms, to limiting lesbian-scene norms. You could write these things on scraps of paper and then burn them together.

* Making a mutual declaration that you are giving up old "games" that hurt the love of both parties.

* Possibly taking off and burning an old piece of clothing as a symbol of "old times."

* If one or both still have "unsettled accounts," performing a short ritual of apology and reconciliation, as well as a mutual promise that these old things will not be brought up again.

2. Tuning in for the couple and the guests

* The guests form two circles, one circle around each of the two women. The guests each share with her the feminine quality they most associate with her. The woman is strengthened by the collective mirroring of all her advantages and good qualities. Then she switches over into the other woman's circle, and the other enters her circle and sits in the middle of it. Qualities central to her partner are embodied by each of the participants, that is, through movement or pantomime, gestures, or even clothing (after a break for getting changed), and finally with a collective dance of these qualities. In this way, she receives, without words, an impression of the possible kinds of qualities she will encounter in her partner. Then she is allowed to ask for explanations and to be pampered by the group to strengthen her, according to her wishes. She is led

back into her old circle, where her partner has been making her own discoveries.

✳ Body painting with body-friendly paints: Each member of the couple has her back painted by two to five women who have come to an agreement based on the woman's instructions. They paint all kinds of symbols representing the things she would like to leave behind. After the paint has dried, her front side is painted with all the things she would like to express and cultivate in this relationship. When both women are finished being painted, they first perform the dance of the symbols on their backs, then the dance of their front sides. Then they perform a dance of integration with each other, one that develops spontaneously when they bring together their front and back qualities. Finally, everyone dances along in a free dance. If nakedness creates discomfort, the two can do the body painting exclusively with each other.

✳ One or two women who radiate calm could help each partner with "ceremonial" dressing.

✳ The partners could give each other a gift, and maybe give a gift to each of the guests as well.

3. Preparation for the main ritual (for more on rituals, see early part of this chapter)

✳ Clean, air out, and heat the room. Burn sage or similar leaves, spread scents, decorate.

✳ Draw a protective circle.

✳ Call upon the powers, the four elements, the compass points, the above and below, and the middle.

✳ Call upon Tara or other helpful beings (e.g., the spirit of your grandmother or other ancestors).

4. Celebration ritual

Again, the following are just a few suggestions to get you started:

✳ Accompanied by singing or recorded music, the couple is led in, if possible from opposite sides of the room into the middle.

✳ The mistress of the ritual brings them together, lays their hands in each other's, symbolically binds their hands with a red cloth, and burns some incense. It doesn't have to be the classic frankincense and myrrh, but essences they have tested out together in advance or that have been chosen by the ritual mistress. Alternatively, she could spray some scent on them. She speaks a few ceremonial words of recognition and admiration for them as a couple.

✳ Then the couple can read a text they have written or each give a short speech, and possibly make mutual promises to each other.

✳ The couple performs a symbolic gift exchange.

✳ They receive good wishes from everyone in the circle.

✳ The mistress leads the group in attuning everyone's hearts. Use a short heart-breathing exercise, for example, or gently sway together to the melodies of Marie Boine or Sheila Chandra, whose CDs can be found in many shops or online.

✳ Now a bit of champagne or another aphrodisiac drink can be given to the beloved, sip by sip by sip, with an honestly meant compliment accompanying each sip. Or the drink can be passed around by the couple to everyone in the circle. Or everyone can participate in the rose ritual (or parts of it), with the couple in the middle of a circle of sensual, spirited guests.

✳ Everyone dances in front of or for the couple and around them.

✳ Make an energy circle with pelvic thrusts directed toward the couple.

✳ Everyone could participate in "Waves of rapture" (see Exercise 50), with their energy directed toward the couple.

✳ Sing a joyful song with toasts or a prerehearsed meditative song like "From You I Receive," by Gila Antara.

✳ Release the powers, elements, beings.

✳ Say the Tara mantra (see Chapter 1).

✳ Honor the place.

❋ Ceremoniously remove the circle.

❋ Officially end the ritual.

5. Reverberation and climax for the couple

❋ Plan an evening meal.

❋ Make toasts to the future; share lesbian jokes and sayings that bring the whole thing back "down to earth."

❋ Share conversation about the ritual experiences, current feelings, organizational aspects of the ceremony.

❋ Free-form dancing for everyone.

❋ During this time, the couple can disappear almost unnoticed to allow themselves a love ritual for just the two of them.

CREATIVE WAYS TO DEAL WITH STUMBLING BLOCKS
The longer a ritual is, the more stumbling blocks can come up along your mutual path. The best way to overcome smaller as well as larger problems is with patience and humor.

VARIATIONS AND SUGGESTIONS
For ceremonies in a community of tantrikas (tantra-experienced or simply sensual, spirited, open women), all kinds of exercises and games from this book could be included in order to intensify the ritual and make it an unforgettable experience for everyone.

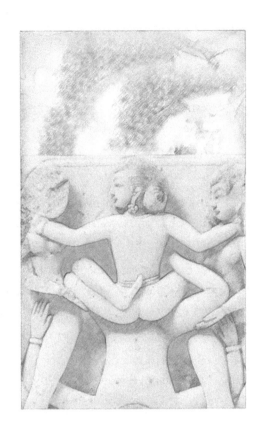

≈ CHAPTER 9 ≈

Games for the Expansion of Love Energy

*A*s I have already mentioned, the main point of what we in the West call tantra is to cultivate our own sensuality, desire, eroticism, and sexuality. Doing so allows us to

* refine all our senses and become more sensitive to ourselves and the world

* strengthen and intensify the pleasures that are presently possible by slowing down external actions and by using the "Six Keys to the Gates of Physical Pleasure" (see Chapter 3, page 55)

* make our encounters with practice partners or love partners more loving, creative, and direct

* strengthen our self-awareness as women in terms of our sexual power and capability of expression, simultaneously improving our autonomy and relationship skills as women

* stop separating out the spiritual dimension of our sexuality, instead fanning our sexual energy so strongly, spreading it out so expansively, and refining its vibrations so carefully that it can be transformed into spiritual energy

The games and exercises introduced in this chapter help prepare your body, soul, and intellect to be fanned into a flame and expanded, whether in the realm of self-love or an encounter with a partner. They can transform the subtly vibrating love energy into an even faster and more subtle energy that "leaves" the material realm.

I myself have joyfully known the sensual experience of dissolving the old patriarchal separation of sexuality and spirituality within me, and of bringing these two parts of my being back together. Spiritual energy is not some "removed" thing, but rather is connected to the earth through our bodies and all their senses.

In order to make the transformation of sexual energy to spiritual energy palpable (for example, in the form of a feeling of deep connection with all living things and belonging in the world; of image and light orgasms; and finally without form, in states of emptiness coming out of fullness), it is worthwhile to prepare your brain just as much as your body to be a space where desire *and* spirituality take place.

🌿 Exercise 46: Fire-breathing orgasm

With this breathing exercise, which may initially seem a little complicated, orgasms can be experienced not as *high points*, but rather as wonderfully orgasmic *high paths*—without any of the usual physical contact. Only with the power of your consciously directed breath can you create arcs of fire that charge up all your chakras and connect them to one another— more powerfully in the lower regions, more tenderly in the upper ones.

GOAL
Reaching an orgasmic state of energy after being purified and after charging the seven main chakras.

TIME AND EXTERNAL PREPARATIONS
About one hour, plus some time to relax after this journey through the depths of your body and soul. If you like to express your feelings by moving, make sure you have enough space to do so. If you like to make sounds, make sure you can do so without a friendly neighbor trying to "help" you.

STEP BY STEP
* Lie down comfortably on your back (without any pillows!) and take several deep, relaxing breaths.

* Visualize and feel how you are drawing earth energy into your first chakra as you breathe in. Fill the root of your being with the life force of your deep inhalation. Remind yourself, here and in the other chakras, of the chakra's characteristics that have been described earlier (see Chapter 2). Give expression to all the feelings that are "stored" in this chakra so that you no longer require the energy to suppress them.

* When the root chakra is completely filled, draw your life energy up to your second chakra, your navel chakra, as you inhale.

* As you exhale, bring your energy back into your first chakra. Become aware of the circular, rocking movements that this creates between the first and second chakras. You might want to imagine a powerful arc of fire that is shooting up within you and flowing back down your front.

✳ Continue with this circular energy motion from the first to the second chakra until the energy there really feels full.

✳ Now enlarge the circle from the first to the third chakra, the solar plexus chakra.

✳ Continue making smaller and larger chakra circles until each chakra feels full: from 1 to 2 and 1 to 3, from 2 to 3 and 2 to 4, from 3 to 4 and 3 to 5, from 4 to 5 and 4 to 6, from 5 to 6 and 5 to 7, from 6 to 7, and finally a really big circle from 7 to 1 and 1 to 7.

✳ If feelings that are waiting to be expressed—and sometimes even unexpected feelings still remaining in the chakras—are "pressed out" while at the same time a high energetic charge connects all the chakras, a feeling of inner satiety, maximal emotional fullness, and pure orgasmic life energy can develop. It can be transformed into peace, stillness, emptiness, or wide open space without any further effort on your part. Here, bliss and emptiness can become one.

✳ Afterward, it is important that you allow yourself a long period of undisturbed peace and meditation (at least thirty minutes; for intense experiences even several hours), so that the awakening fire energy can spread through you in more and more subtle flames.

CREATIVE WAYS TO DEAL WITH STUMBLING BLOCKS

✳ If the energy builds up too strongly in your chest, let it flow out upward by leaning your head back. It can be useful to make sounds so that the energy is not blocked by the throat chakra.

✳ If you have problems building up energy, it can help to return to the first chakra and start over again.

✳ Don't worry if you don't get it "right" on the first try. This is a very strong healing process for your body, and there may be energy blockages that your body needs to dissolve before the energy can flow freely and orgasmically.

VARIATIONS AND SUGGESTIONS

* ✳ Take your time and be patient. You don't need to feel anything special, but you can notice everything and don't have to push anything away.

* ✳ Although you are continually making smaller and larger circles to connect the chakras, let a continual flow of energy move from the first chakra (possibly supported by a pumping of the PC muscle) to the uppermost chakra, and focus on that.

* ✳ If possible, practice several times a week. Soon you will be able to let the flow of the fire breathing happen spontaneously.

* ✳ If both you and your partner want to, you can do this sequence in the "bonding" position, lying one on top of the other with stomachs touching (see illustration below). The person on top lays her head on a small pillow next to the lower partner's head. You only touch foreheads when focusing on the two uppermost chakras. So that you can coordinate, the person on the bottom determines when you will move to the next chakra circle, tapping with her fingers on her partner's back to indicate the location of each new

**Figure 6.
The bonding
position.**

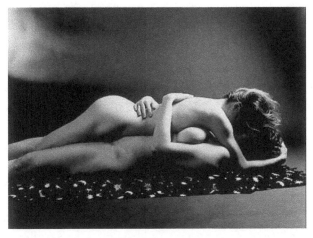

chakra. You should switch before it gets uncomfortable for either. In any case, an enormous orgiastic energy can develop between the two of you—but only through your mutual "panting"!

🐚 Exercise 47: Rosette-rose massage

This is a pelvic-floor healing massage for women that is especially effective when repeated several times. For many women it will clearly be an advanced exercise, since it requires placing yourself, with all the sensitivity and vulnerability of an opened anus, in the loving hands of another person. In addition, the yoni is touched from within, which requires great openness with your partner.

GOAL

Freeing the entire root chakra (from the anus to the yoni) from blockages and other old patterns of pain. This creates one of the most important conditions for the free flow of love energy.

TIME AND EXTERNAL PREPARATIONS

About two hours per partner, with enough time for discussion and for a break before switching. Preparation of a particularly nice love nest, possibly with power objects, flowers, and beautiful personal objects at the head; a blanket or cloth at the ready for the phase of introspection; two glasses of water and maybe a little tray with paper towels, massage oil, Vaseline (better for the sensitive inner skin of the anus than water-soluble lubricants, since the oil base creates a stronger protective layer; it does also reduce sensitivity, so it's not ideal for the yoni!); possibly a water-based lubricant (for the skin around the anus, since the water base keeps pores open; also, it's better for anal dildos, should you decide to use them later); finger cots or latex gloves for easier movement, safer sex, and to avoid unpleasant feelings at the thought of coming into contact with fecal matter; disinfectant for additional disinfecting of fingers after the massage; peppermint water to neutralize any unpleasant-seeming smells. *The active partner, or "pleasure companion," needs to thoroughly trim and file her fingernails ahead of time.*

STEP BY STEP

* First, make eye contact and tune in to each other in a loud way; for example, by dancing to drum music or performing the "Dance of the she-demons" (Exercise 22).

✳ Then the recipient may express any wishes and fears or give information, and the companion can pose any last questions.

✳ *If you're the pleasure companion,* bless the recipient's three main chakras (first the root chakra, then the heart, and finally the third eye). Do this by touching each chakra in turn, with your eyes closed, as you try to find the appropriate sensual-flowery words of honor and respect to awaken it through the power of the spirit.

✳ After undressing, the recipient lies down slowly on her belly, and the pleasure companion sits down on the recipient's left side. (If you are left-handed, you should sit on the recipient's right side.)

✳ *Pleasure companion,* rub your hands together in order to energize them, and begin to touch the sacrum and the rear heart chakra with your warm hands. After a moment of calm, begin to shake or vibrate them a little, and then begin to put your weight on the larger muscles of the back, buttocks, and legs.

✳ Now, using some massage oil, begin a short back massage, emphasizing the large muscles of the back, the buttocks, the thighs, and the calves.

✳ Take a moment to assure the recipient, without words, that she is in good hands with you—for example, by holding her soles calmly and firmly for a few breaths.

✳ Then sit down next to the recipient so that you can comfortably reach her anus, and slowly begin to pull the recipient's buttocks apart, touching the area above the "rosette," or sphincter, with your fingertips, your thumb, or even your knuckles.

✳ Circle directly around the rosette and gently stretch its skin outward, as though you were carefully trying to stroke the innermost petals of a flower.

✳ When the recipient is ready, put on a finger cot or a well-fitting latex glove, rub it with Vaseline, and lay your finger gently on the rosette. You can continue to circle, too, and if the recipient is highly sensitive or fears injury, you can spread a little Vaseline or other lubricant on the whole anal area.

✳ Do not force your way in, but let yourself, when the time is right, be pulled into the anus by small sucking motions on the recipient's part. Stay there a moment so that the recipient can adjust to this feeling.

✳ *Recipient,* from now on, use mostly your voice and your hands to expresses any feelings that come up during the rosette or anus massage. Since there are often painful emotions, it is important that you not pull away quickly or tell your companion to remove her finger; instead, ask your companion to find a finger position that allows you to relax into the emotional hurt or to express it in such a way that it can dissolve. (This really works, as long as the recipient of these strange pleasures breathes deeply enough.)

✳ Now, *pleasure companion,* moving very carefully and a millimeter at a time, begin to stretch the outer rosette, the first of two in the anus, in all directions possible from this position.

✳ If you reach a physically or emotionally painful spot, do not jerk back with your finger as soon as the pain is expressed; instead, wait calmly or "ring" the anus a little or just take away some of the pressure, so that the recipient has a chance to relax and breathe into the pain or to express any painful emotions. Wait until the recipient is ready for new experiences again and is able to return to the expectation and experiencing of pleasure.

✳ *Recipient,* if you let your companion's finger farther inside, the companion now stretches the anus to both sides, toward the sit bones (particularly toward the sitting bone on the side where the companion is seated). If this is painful, you can experiment with consciously clenching your buttocks and firmly saying or yelling *no.* (Here, as in every phase of the massage, you as the recipient have the power to decide if you want to stop immediately—for example, if the pain is not lessened simply by breathing or if old traumatic experiences surface that would be better dealt with in a therapeutic context rather than in this sort of massage.)

✳ *Companion,* use your other hand to touch the other chakras repeatedly, laying it on the rear navel or heart chakra, for example. Continue to communicate with the recipient throughout the whole massage, so that you can recognize even tiny expressions of pleasure or displeasure and adjust your massage accordingly.

✳ The second, inner rosette is stretched just like the first one.

✳ The coccyx (tailbone) can be touched from the inside; it's a good idea, though, to hold your thumb against it from the outside, because the projection of the coccyx is very sensitive and often needs a point of resistance.

✳ The kundalini point, lying at the end of the coccyx, can be massaged as well, which often creates strong feelings of desire. Here, too, it is important to make sure the recipient can express whatever feelings come up.

✳ If you feel tender spots of gravel-like tissue with your finger, it is often a good idea to linger there, unless the recipient does not want you to.

✳ *Recipient,* if you find the need to feel more of your own power (rather than, say, getting mired in childish feelings of helplessness), you can get up on all fours and move your hips spontaneously.

✳ After doing that, you can gradually turn over onto your back by turning toward the companion with your right leg lifted; the companion sits between your legs, leaving their finger(s) in your anus during the turning process.

✳ Now look at each other for a moment and exchange a small nicety or compliment about the process so far; the recipient now has another chance to express any wishes.

✳ Next, *pleasure companion,* touch the recipient's chakras from the front, and as you proceed, continue to connect them with each other through occasional small massages or caresses, so that the root chakra is not dealt with in isolation.

* Now the first rosette, then the second, and then the other sit bone and the broader tunnel on the other side (the vagina) are stretched with movements like those used in the belly position. It is very important here to make eye contact for every feeling expressed and, if necessary, to use words to discuss the recipient's wishes and boundaries. The pleasure companion tries to act on the recipient's wishes as precisely as possible so that the recipient can experience being the order-giver, even in such a passive position.

* Then, *companion,* tap on the perineum a few times to activate the pelvic muscle.

* After doing that, take a second finger cot or glove, put lubricant on it, and find your way slowly through your partner's pleasure forest to the gate of the yoni. It is important that you *never* use the same finger to visit the yoni, even after using a disinfectant (unless you have changed gloves or finger cots), because it will probably react angrily to the rectal bacteria and become infected! Here, too, you should not force your way in actively, but rather let yourself be "sucked in," moving very carefully and stretching the vagina in every conceivable direction.

* Then the fingers in the anus and the vagina can move together like scissors, thoroughly massaging the wall between them. Supported by the recipient's deep breathing, this tissue can (finally, for once) relax and enjoy better circulation; the massage leaves the recipient with a feeling of breadth and depth in the root area.

* Then the first finger can be slowly drawn out of the anus while the vaginal finger carefully, with good communication between the recipient and the companion, feels for the G-spot and presses, circles, or strokes it a little. The opening of the uterus, too, that arched "end" of the yoni tunnel with the little slit, can be thoroughly massaged. However, the companion should make sure not to massage the opening too much, but all around it instead.

✳ Sometimes, for example while the pubic bone is being massaged from the inside, it can be nice when light pressure is applied from outside. If massive emotions (for example, memory fragments of rape or abuse situations) make themselves felt, it's important to make sure the recipient is not overwhelmed; the spots should only be touched enough to let the feelings be expressed. (The use of the recipient's voice and possibly even concrete words can be more important here than spontaneous physical reactions.)

✳ If more and more feelings of desire come up, the recipient can breathe deeply into them to balance out a little of the stress of working through the pain.

✳ While the companion continues to leave a finger in the vagina, both partners begin to breathe heavily together, and the recipient might support the sexual breathing through pelvic movements.

✳ Then the pleasure companion carefully pulls the finger out of the vagina, takes off the glove or finger cot, and sits up more comfortably, if necessary.

✳ Now, *recipient,* you go into the "big draw." That is, as you inhale, powerfully draw all your energy upward: Close your anus, tense all your muscles and especially close your throat chakra, and remain in this state as long as you can while holding your breath. When you feel like you can't hold your breath any longer, pull a last little bit of air in through the crown chakra and then let go of yourself and everything else, giving in to spontaneous movements, images, etc.

✳ *Pleasure companion,* breathe with the recipient for a little while longer, then retreat a bit, cover the recipient up if she wants to be covered, and remain connected to the recipient without touching her. (During this time, only background music should be played. You might select something from the category "For resonating," listed in Resources.)

✳ If the recipient doesn't want to lie alone, both of you can cuddle and spend some time together in peaceful silence.

✳ After this, without changing position, briefly discuss the experience.

✳ Conclude with a heart-to-heart embrace (see Exercise 25).

✳ In the time following the massage, *recipient,* you are often very open and sensitive, so you should find ways to protect yourself, determining what degree of closeness or distance you need, etc.

✳ *Pleasure companion,* you may be somewhat exhausted, and you should ideally shower to wash out of your body the excess energy you have absorbed. A trip to the sauna might be good, too.

CREATIVE WAYS TO DEAL WITH STUMBLING BLOCKS

✳ Women who have been sexually traumatized, have undergone traumatic birthing experiences, or have had a rigid sanitary upbringing sometimes carry various blockages and physical memories away from these experiences. The feelings that arise during the massage need to be expressed (through moaning or screaming, etc.). If the feelings are so intense that they cannot be released in this way, the woman receiving the massage should not feel she must endure it. She could ask her companion for other kinds of touches, like a comforting hand on her belly and forehead or whatever she might need to provide a healing alternative to the memories of old hurts that are surfacing.

✳ If the exercise is very pleasurable (perhaps surprisingly so) for the recipient, but she is trying to forbid this feeling ("yuck, how dirty/indecent!"), the companion can help by encouraging her to give her silent pleasure a voice or to give in to movements. Or, *companion,* you can tell her, by way of honest compliments, how glad you are that you can provide her with this pleasure.

✳ Some recipients project their inner taboos outward and are afraid of posing a challenge for their partners. Here I can only share my experience that it can be a distinct pleasure for women with a highly sanitary upbringing to have the distance between joy and shit pleasurably shrink down to zero.

✳ However, please don't feel any new "pleasure stress"! The first massage of this kind may be too strange, the second too painful, the third more frightening than pleasurable, but then... and then...!

VARIATIONS AND SUGGESTIONS

If the recipient would prefer to receive, say, just the rosette massage without the yoni contact (or vice versa), her companion acts accordingly, of course, and only touches that entrance.

🐚 Exercise 48: MMM: Magic "mussel" massage

For me, the magic "mussel" (yoni) massage is the heart and soul of tantra for women! It is never the same and never has the same effect from one time to the next, but it has always shown me important facets of my desire. It is wonderfully suited to the deepening and freshening up of sexuality between lovers but can also be done with someone you know less well as long as your sympathies and your playfulness match up well and you are considerate with each other.

We are playing with the following components: increased consciousness through touching, fanning desire, spreading this energy through the whole body, and bundling it together for a transcendental experience. Breathing plays a large role—both parties should keep breathing deeply, quickly, and consciously.

The massage is divided into two parts, each with a "big draw" as the grand finale. Since, in general, women have access to their *entire* bodies as erotic instruments of pleasure, this massage consciously addresses the entire body as an erogenous zone. Only in the last phase do stronger "yoni grips" come into play.

GOAL

According to Taoist philosophy, this massage creates energy. Specifically, it creates *ching chi,* or sexually colored, fast, and expansive life energy. *Ching chi* can be felt in sensations of desire, vitality, and vibration. In a resting state, the *ching chi* is connected with the organs and muscles of the root and navel chakras; with the "MMM," it is spread throughout the whole body. The mussel massage is supported by heart breathing (clear, powerful inhalation into the heart region) and its temporary combination with a quick tensing of the PC muscle. The combination of heart breathing and "MMM" can climax in a full-body orgasm (a high level of charge with simultaneous deep relaxation).

Still, an orgasm is not the goal, but rather an orgasmic or orgiastic (joyfully aroused and simultaneously relaxed) state reached by connecting breath-charging and the freed-up *ching chi*.

TIME AND EXTERNAL PREPARATIONS

At least an hour (or two if possible) to avoid time pressure. Set up a warm, pleasant, undisturbed, not-too-full room with a beautiful, soft bed; prepare your own body by showering, applying lotion, jewelry, etc. Inner preparations: You may want to participate in a mood-setting transition ritual (see Exercise I), a silent meditation (done together or individually), a greeting, a discussion of wishes and boundaries, and a loving acknowledgment of the current mood and feelings of the other person.

STEP BY STEP

Instructions for the enjoyer

* Submit actively to your pleasure companion and her hands without "becoming an object"; that is, acknowledge that *you yourself,* and not your companion's activities, are responsible for your pleasure.

* Play with the "six keys to the gates of physical pleasure" (see Chapter 3, page 55): deep breathing, spontaneous movement, sounds and tones, concentration and consciousness, playing in the moment, practice and habit.

* Give in to all of your feelings and impulses—express them and look inside yourself again. Remember, arousal usually comes in waves. Let go of your expectations of how arousal should be expressed. You don't need to do anything except breathe deeply and continually return to your physical sensations. In the last phase, you don't even need to do that; you only have to give in to your momentary state of being.

✳ If you don't like something, or you have requests for your pleasure companion, express them lovingly and clearly, or share them with gestures or sounds.

✳ Relax more and more into your arousal, and enjoy every second of your life.

Instructions for the companion

✳ Let yourself be guided by your intuition, without trying to reach a particular goal. Let go of your fears of any kind of failure. Replace technical skill with heartfelt feeling, and trust in your sensitivity. Don't hide your uncertainty behind the "heating up" of desire, and leave your partner time and space for the beautiful, joyous, earthy vibrations that she can give you.

✳ Allow your partner and yourself the pleasure of slow, intense touches.

✳ You are giving your partner a journey, and in the process you can arrive at yourself. Grant yourself this wonderful experience of female power as your partner blooms under your hands and dissolves into pure joy.

Instructions for both

I. Coming into the body

✳ This can be accompanied by a mutually passionate or very cautious undressing, as well as playful shows of strength and a warm-up massage for the recipient that might include the following:

 — stroking the whole body with your fingertips, caressing and massaging her

 — if you know them, pressing the acupressure points on her fingertips and the tips of her toes

 — powerfully massaging the inner thigh, belly, and back muscles

 — gently massaging the forehead, nose, ears, cheeks, lips, neck, and head

— using both hands simultaneously to massage her breasts in a circular motion (from the middle upward and around, or the reverse)

— and finally, rubbing her with coconut oil. The oil should be nice and warm, and it should be sprayed very generously from a bottle onto the backs of your hands, which are used for the oil application. The advantage of coconut oil is its thinness—it slides unexpectedly well.

✳ *Pleasure companion,* what is important here is your ability to do two different things at once with your left hand (the heart-hand) and your right hand (the yoni-hand; lefties can, of course, switch hands): While the yoni-hand awakens energy (in the whole belly-pelvis-thigh area), the heart-hand distributes it, mainly throughout the upper body; the lower torso, legs, and feet are partially included too. The distribution of energy with the heart-hand makes it possible for the whole body to take in the *ching chi,* or sex energy. In this way it becomes possible to store much more energy than in conventional genital sex, since without distribution there would simply be a discharge of energy. The recipient contributes to the creation and distribution of energy with her "heart-breathing."

✳ Heart-mussel touching: Place one hand on the mussel (yoni) and the other on the heart of the recipient. The mussel-hand can lie there calmly, while the other hand connects the heart and mussel through massage.

✳ Then the enjoyer lies down on her back, and you touch her much more erotically all over the body—with fingers, feathers, and furs, with hair and hot breath, with moist lips, and, above all, with a lot of playful imagination and a lot of time "spread out" over her body. Think about stretching out the enjoyer's body: Take her fingers and toes and massage them while pulling on them; pull her hair gently upward with your fingers, like a comb. Then scratch her yoni-forest and tug on the yoni-forest hair. In this phase, adjust your breathing to that of the recipient so it remains attuned to her.

An important element is making sounds together, which sets energy in motion.

* Then comes the first gentle "big draw" (see Exercise 47).

* This warm-up massage can be made shorter or longer depending on your familiarity with each other and your capacity for devotion. The important thing is that you satisfy the recipient! Satisfy her body with gentle, powerful, tender touches! Look for signs of well-being on the recipient's part and for her readiness to move on to the next phase.

2. Sexual peaking

In this phase, sexual energy is first coaxed out of various places; the "flames" are fanned and then distributed. Then the flames are bundled together and distributed even more subtly and transformed into quick vibrating energy on a subtle, material level. The pleasure companion can sit between the recipient's legs for this part. Here are some suggestions for individual steps:

Sneaking up from the outside

* Egg-warming: Rub your hands together, charge them up, and run them gently over the ovaries (from the outside).

* Uterus warming: Your left hand covers the mussel, and the right strokes the uterus (from the outside) in a circular motion.

* Uterus drumroll: Use your fingertips to drum with quick, light slaps on her lower belly, at the level of the uterus, and her inner thighs.

* Greeting the G-spot: Carefully dig and press your fingers into the outer belly region, around the bladder and G-spot—slowly, powerfully, gently, and deeply.

* Spinning top, or vulva vibration: The whole hand covers the vulva and vibrates deeply into it; the other hand, vibrating, goes from chakra to chakra or at least to the heart chakra. Meanwhile, hum or even growl to strengthen the feeling of a "slightly tipsy yoni."

* Pussy petting: Your well-oiled hands gently tap on the whole mussel region (the inner thighs, the belly region, and from the coccyx to the mons veneris).

* Stroll in the forest: The yoni hair is scratched and tugged, particularly around the smaller labia.

* Tap dance of the quick hands: Your fingertips and maybe even palms tap and knock on the vulva and clitoris.

Most of these activities are less about targeting arousal than about having a relaxing, exciting, or consciousness-raising effect and are also about making it easier for the enjoyer to allow herself to give in to even more touches.

Flirting with the mussel's inner life

Pleasure companion, from this phase on, it is usually more comfortable to sit *next to* the recipient. It is important for you to be comfortable, so that you avoid massaging any of your own physical tension into the recipient or ruining your own fun. If you don't know each other very well, a few words about needs and boundaries are always a good idea.

* Pouty lips: Press the outer and inner labia together with your fingers, and massage them.

* Zig-zag lips: Push the lips against each other with your thumbs.

* Lip-shiatsu: If you know them, press the shiatsu points between the inner and outer labia slowly and—if the recipient wishes—at times even forcefully.

* Tour de France: Use your fingertips to circle all the way around the inner labia up to the clitoris and back, at a quick tempo.

* Pussy-push: Press the outer labia together with your index fingers and pull them upward as though they were about to lift off.

* Light my fire: Surround the mussel with both hands, and rub the labia together as if you were starting a fire.

✳ Butterfly: Open and close the mussel with both hands, using your fingers to playfully unfold, close, and unfold the labia again. As you open them, blow warm air into them.

✳ Opening the mussel: Your thumbs and index fingers press, pull, and massage the inner and outer labia upward, downward, and to the sides.

✳ Knocking at the yoni-gate: Knock on the door by gently laying your index finger on the opening and waiting for the recipient to pulse her PC muscle, indicating that she is ready to draw it in.

✳ The four compass points: If possible, use a second finger to gently but firmly widen the entrance to the mussel in all directions, pausing for a second at each compass point. If, for example, a slight burning or pulling occurs to the "south," do not simply pull your finger away, but let it remain, exerting gentle pressure. The recipient first breathes powerfully, then more gently, while concentrating on this spot, and makes sounds until the pain slowly dissolves into warmth or other sensations. Only then do you continue. The recipient decides whether she can deal with or dissolve any pain that may arise, or whether this spot should not be touched anymore.

✳ Spelunking: As you did with the four compass points, explore every spot in the pleasure cave. Be on a constant search for pleasure spots or pain spots, making the recipient aware of them and helping her express and dissolve them. Clear words can be important here, particularly in spots near the bones and bladder.

✳ First one, then two, then three, then many: Enter the mussel with as many fingers as the recipient wants to take in, and move them as gently or vigorously as the recipient likes.

Fanning the flame of the pearl

✳ Rock around the clitoris: The left thumb and index finger open the mussel, while the right index finger circles around the pearl (clitoris).

* Hat on, hat off: Use your thumb and index finger to pull the hood (the little hat) forward and back.

* Knocking on heaven's door: Knock and ring or vibrate on the pearl mound (very few women prefer this directly on the clitoris).

* Plucking pearls: Play around, twirling and rubbing the clitoris and its little hood between your thumb and index finger.

* Polishing the pearl: Pull the hood back with the thumb and finger of your right hand, and massage the clitoris directly from above or from the side, on its stem or its root (not every recipient likes to have her clitoris directly stimulated).

* Grasping the stem from the root to the blossom: Rub the shaft of the clitoris—especially along the sides—between the hood and root, at the beginning of the labia, and emphasize its length in your movements.

Flames from all directions

* Glowing fire with jets of flame: Sit on the recipient's left side. With your left hand under her coccyx, your thumb pulls the mussel entrance a little in the direction of the anus. Your right hand lies on her pubic bone, and your thumb and index finger gently massage the pearl as described above, slowly increasing the speed and maybe the intensity as well.

* Waxing moon: Your left thumb reaches as far as possible into the lust-tunnel and turns slowly until your left hand is on top. Then the pearl can be pressed with the ball of your hand while your fingertips continue to press and vibrate the outer G-spot with each exhalation.

* Three-in-one: Sit sideways. With your left hand under the coccyx, use your thumb to pull the mussel entrance toward the anus. Your right hand lies on your partner's mons veneris, and you switch off between massaging the pearl with the ball of your hand and massaging the outside of the G-spot with your fingertips. If the recipient can give up control and precise perception in order to

submit openly to her companion's game and to her own pleasure, she can have heavenly experiences in the active worship of her yoni.

Liquefying the flame within

* Surrounding and ringing (vibrating) the goddess-point: Both of you find the G-spot together, which the pleasure companion then massages in various ways. Use powerful pressing and releasing, rubbing, ringing, and simultaneous massage from the inside (left hand) and the outside (right hand). The enjoyer can pump with her PC muscle during this process. She does "push-outs" (that is, pushes her pelvis muscle outward). If she is extremely aroused, this can result in an ejaculation (pleasure fountain).

* Ringing the U-spot: Vibrating, pressing, rubbing, or circling around the urinary tract's erectile tissue, which lies close to the urethra, can cause a special bean-shaped spot of erectile tissue to emerge. Stimulating it, like stimmulating the G-spot, can result in an ejaculation.

* Calling upon the primordial mother: When the recipient's pelvic floor is relaxed, massage the mouth of her uterus with two fingers of your left hand, while the other hand holds the uterus from the outside.

* Light vibration on the M-spot: You usually can only find this point when the recipient is highly aroused. It lies in the vaginal roof that often forms only after a first orgasm and is made up of the walls of the vagina and uterus. It can be lightly vibrated or just gently touched, and it helps to develop a sweet, hot lava flow in an upward direction, triggering the tendency toward more implosive orgasms.

* Twist and shout: One or more fingers twist around in the recipient's love tunnel, vigorously push into it, or circle around near the gate. The pleasure companion twists, and the recipient shouts or makes other sounds of pleasure.

* Pause and silence: Both partners remain motionless while the fingers rest inside the mussel.

* Continue however the recipient likes: Ask her what she'd like the best. Some recipients like a specific order when you are caressing the pleasure centers or would like to be kissed on their Venus-lips and to have their pearl and yoni-entrance licked. (A wonderful, subtle vibration is usually experienced if the companion hums while she is doing this).

3. Leading into the mountaintop experience

This has to do with playing around the edge of an orgasm.

* Try the "stop" technique: Every time the enjoyer has almost reached the *point of no return*—that is, she is just short of reaching an explosive orgasm—she gives a signal to stop.

* The pleasure companion pauses for a few seconds and then continues the massage until the recipient once again reaches this point of arousal and says, "Stop!" It is a good idea to try to reach the point of no return at least three times in thirty minutes without going past it (peaking).

* While peaking, the recipient can tense her PC muscle and draw her energy up through the inner flute (see Exercise 16), through the heart, and into the third eye.

* For a variation, try the "9-1" rhythm: Massage the clitoris nine times with the recipient's favorite motion, skip one beat, again massage nine times, skip a beat, etc. Continue, depending on how fast the recipient can become aroused again and how quickly or slowly she usually glides into an orgasm.

* For another variation, switch off between the clitoris and the G-spot, for example spend ten seconds at the clitoris and ten seconds at the G-spot (or other spots). For the greatest pleasure, timing needs to be determined by good communication and a little intuition. What is important is that the recipient is able to build up arousal without discharging it orgasmically and without having any control over this rhythm.

4. Distributing pleasure in all directions

This "all-around ecstasy" can occur when the coaxed-out sexual energy is spread throughout the body, bundled up as much as possible, and then transformed during a phase of silence.

* Distributing: Distribute the energy from the enjoyer's root chakra through her whole body with a gentle breath or a feather-light hand, particularly emphasizing the vertical direction.

* Closing the gates: Close her lower gates (labia and anus) with your hand, and let your hand rest there for a moment while you breathe along with the recipient. You might also close her upper gates— ears, eyes, and nose—with the fingers of your other hand.

* "Big draw": The recipient draws in all the energy available to her with a deep breath and a pumping of the PC muscle, pulling the energy up to the heart region, the third eye, or the crown chakra. Then she holds her breath as long as she can. She closes all her openings, particularly the area around the throat chakra, tenses all her muscles as much as she can, and takes one last little breath toward the crown chakra before she exhales. As she exhales, she lets go of all her tension, in her sphincter muscles in particular, and gives in to any physical sensations, spontaneous movements, feelings, and image worlds that come up.

* Variation with emphasis on the heart: The recipient chooses a point in time when she will catch a wave of pleasure. When the wave comes, she takes about twenty "heart-breaths" and then three deep breaths toward her pelvic floor. During this time she can let herself be given a couple more fiery impulses—for example, on her pearl. Then the pleasure companion removes her hands, and the recipient tenses all the muscles in her body as tightly as she can. The result is that her upper body and legs lift up slightly, and all her energy is pressed deep inside her. There it shoots upward through delicate channels. In a body that is free of major blockages, this enormous charge will push consciousness into a realm where separation is replaced by connection, and silence and peace are able to spread out.

✳ Caretaking and silence: Wrap the enjoyer up in a blanket and make sure that she can be left alone and undisturbed (with nonrhythmic background music or complete silence in the room).

✳ In this phase, very different methods of transforming energy can become possible—for example, a deeply touching feeling of devoted love for yourself, for the other, for the whole world; or a clear and natural feeling of connection with all living beings; or visions of love lived without hindrances; or many brightly colored pictures, sounds, or atmospheres; or an exciting "home theater" in your head with films about flying or romantic encounters or creative acts; or, or, or.... All of this occurs only occasionally and is rarely noticeable from the outside; sometimes a smile or a slight vibration can be detected, but sometimes the recipient just seems to be sleeping. These tantric ecstasies spread out most effectively in meditative silence, during extended periods of time, and in the loving, attentive presence of the partner, even if that person's presence is occasionally forgotten.

✳ Exchange and lying together: The recipient is allowed to determine the type of contact here.

✳ Conclude with a heart-to-heart embrace or some other clearly defined ending to the ritual.

🦢 Exercise 49: Ecstatic mountaintop experiences

This exercise deals with extended sexual orgasm, also known as extended super orgasm, or ESO. ESO is a deep orgasm lasting thirty minutes or longer. My teacher Margot Anand terms it *MORe* (multiorgasmic response). During an ESO, the spiritual dimension of sexual happiness can be experienced on the various energy levels. The basis for the experience can be the "MMM" (Exercise 48).

Physically speaking, the muscle contractions involved in an orgasm can be described as follows:

✳ Surface contractions: These occur during a "normal" orgasm. They are involuntary contractions of the PC muscle, usually brought about by stimulation of the clitoris, that may feel as though the perineum and the lower third of the vagina are contracting about once per second.

✳ Deep contractions: Here, the musculature of the upper third of the vagina and of the uterus contracts; it causes "push-outs" of the deep pelvic muscles that can last ten seconds or longer.

✳ If the deeper contractions are mixed with surface contractions, the feeling of pleasure increases, reaches a plateau, increases again, etc. We will refer to this as phase 1 ESO.

✳ If lasting, slow push-outs replace the mixed contractions, and each lasts up to thirty seconds, this is what we will refer to as phase 2 ESO.

GOAL

Using your hand and/or mouth, you will lead the enjoyer to orgasmic ecstasies in which sexual energy becomes spiritual. She no longer has climaxes or "high points," but inwardly traverses extended "high paths." The experience can create an orgasmic feeling for life, lasting longer than these kinds of exercises, founded in the trust that you are "in the hands of something greater," and it creates that famous sex appeal in your encounters with others.

TIME AND EXTERNAL PREPARATIONS

At least two hours. Prepare everything else as for the "MMM" (Exercise 48).

STEP BY STEP

✳ After a warm-up phase, such as that described in step 1 of the "MMM," various ways of stroking the clitoris are recommended. (Basically, all the kinds of touching described in the "MMM" can be used here.) Stroke the clitoris indirectly or slowly and regularly (once per second) for several minutes. Use plenty of lubricant, because of the length of the massage. Change your stroke only gradually, paying attention to signs of increased arousal (the yoni growing larger and darker, sounds, movements, pushing against your hand, sweating, the pearl swelling and drawing downward or inward toward the vagina).

* When the enjoyer is just about to reach orgasm, the surface contractions of her pelvic-floor muscle may begin. At this point, switch to stimulating the vagina. Do this by stretching the vaginal walls, moving your fingers or tongue in and out, or—best— vibrating the G-spot. Right now—just before an orgasm (as well as just after)—this spot is pain-free, pleasure-filled, and easy to feel (see Chapter 2 for a description of how to find the G-spot), and it can be stimulated with slow, strong pressure. Or try "ring- ing" it by pressing it softly, but in a sustained way. This inner stimulation creates a stronger contraction of the vaginal muscles than the stimulation of the clitoris; the uterine muscles and the rear third of the vagina contract as well.

* In a "normal" orgasm, the vagina grows longer and pulls upward toward the belly (tenting). Meanwhile, your finger might easily lose contact with the G-spot. Tenting indicates climax or orgasm—a plateau in ESO phase I. In later phases it indicates approaching resistance.

* During tenting, stimulate the G-spot more gently and slowly, and return to the clitoris until the recipient reacts with PC contrac- tions and push-outs again; then return to the G-spot. Switching off between clitoris and G-spot (or sometimes simultaneously stimulating the two) causes arousal to increase until it reaches another plateau (pause, resistance, etc.). This can take about fifteen minutes (phase I of the ESO). Various factors determine the intensity and frequency of the push-outs here: (1) speed, pressure, and placement of the stimulating finger, and (2) the recipient's capacity to trust and her ability to let go of resistance.

* And now for the most important phase: *For the enjoyer,* this means taking her time and doing absolutely nothing. Only when she completely lets go and gives up control can she enjoy lasting, soft, long waves of deep push-out contractions, accompanied by

the further stimulation of the clitoris and G-spot. This is phase 2 of the ESO, experienced as timelessness, melting, high arousal, and reduced pulse and blood pressure, the ability to become aroused again and reach orgasm very quickly, along with image- and light-ecstasies, etc.—in short, a timeless pleasure and deep happiness.

CREATIVE WAYS TO DEAL WITH STUMBLING BLOCKS

✳ When someone is already very open but has not yet relaxed into her arousal enough to become flowing, she is very susceptible to distractions of every kind. The only thing that helps here is smart management of distractions (see Chapter 3) as well as a sense of humor on both sides.

✳ If the recipient does let herself fall into a regular orgasm during this exercise, it doesn't matter; it will just take a little longer to build up again to the appropriate level of arousal. So don't allow any stress that could come from a no orgasm policy! Instead, pay loving attention to every detail of the paths taken by pleasure.

VARIATIONS AND SUGGESTIONS

Sometimes, consciously slowing down each touch can create more depth and intensity for the recipient and, along with occasional eye contact, can create more closeness for both.

🐟 Exercise 50: Waves of rapture

This is a method of happiness developed by Margot Anand wherein the energy received from love-play or transformed by the "MMM" or ESO is shared with the other person in a quiet, touching way, so that both feel as if they were in flight or as if they were connected like the ebb and flow of a broad ocean. They may even meet beyond the borders of their personalities. Here, sexual fire becomes water—"firewater." And if your body is open enough, the waves will spread through all your bodily fluids, through all the cells, letting the released endorphins (happiness hormones) unfold their gratifying effects. This can be physically experienced as a vibration and flowing of delicate energy streams through all levels of the body.

Emotionally, feelings of love, happiness, and peace spread out, and mentally there develops an impression of spacelessness and timelessness, of the eternity of the moment.

However, the "wave" can also be practiced without any preliminary sexual charging—just for fun—for example, when both people feel good together and just want to enjoy each other quietly.

GOAL

By sitting together in the melting position (see yab-yum, Exercise 33), with chakras aligned, two people can achieve an exponential increase of energies. This can occur on the level of the individual chakras as well. A quiet joy is experienced together; an indescribable source of power for your everyday life.

TIME AND EXTERNAL PREPARATIONS

After massages like the "MMM" or ESO, take at least half an hour or a whole hour of quiet time for the two of you. The amount of time you allow will depend on your physical ability to sit in the yab-yum for long periods of time.

STEP BY STEP

* After sex together (or as a silent exercise), sit in the yab-yum, the melting position. One person sits on the floor with legs crossed (if possible, without a cushion), and the other sits upright in the first person's lap, facing her, with legs around her hips. *If you're the person on top,* it is a good idea to slide slowly into the other's lap. You can begin with your arms behind you as support and then slowly lower your weight onto your partner. First, your weight is supported by the soles of your feet, then by your calves, then by your thighs. Imagine being connected with the sky as you touch your soles to each other behind the other's rump. Begin by supporting each other with your hands on each other's backs, at the coccyx and the rear heart chakra, so that you both receive an impulse to sit up straight.

* Now you, *as the person sitting on top,* close your eyes, and begin to move your pelvis; let it dance forward and backward and let it

circle. Play with different images: You are making love to yourself, you are an African goddess, or you imagine that a big snake is uncoiling inside you. Once you have felt yourself, open your eyes. Take notice of your yoni, your perineum, your rump; let them take part in your movement. You become seductive, trying out smaller and larger pelvic circles. Imagine that you are sitting in the crotch of a tree and are being moved by the wind. Let the clown, the child, the witch, the goddess in you, the Shakti or Tara, play.

✳ *As the person sitting on the bottom,* you are like the earth, resting or shaking. You also move your pelvis in your own way, moving the other person along with you. It is important for both of you to let your movements come from your centers. (If you "go limp" at some point in this position, you can restart your energy by propping your arms behind you and moving that way for a while. Afterward, return to the yab-yum position again. In fact, you can take occasional breaks throughout, rather than letting the person on the bottom forget the earthy qualities of her being because her feet have fallen asleep.) Allow yourself to feel the strength of the earth's power. When breathing in unison, you set the tone.

✳ As the movement continues, you both include your PC muscles (tense, release, push down, and play with various rhythms).

✳ Add sexual breathing. When you pull your pelvis back, tense the PC muscle, take the energy in, and breathe in. As your pelvis rolls forward, relax and breathe out. This is similar to the chakra wave or the fire-breathing orgasm, in which you guide your fire upward through all the chakras.

✳ You create your energetic field, imagining that your ideal image of the inner beloved (see Exercise 10) is combining with your real beloved, who is not just a person with strengths and weaknesses, but also an embodiment of, for example, the goddess Tara.

✳ Now try to establish a common rhythm in your pelvic rocking. Lay one hand on your partner's coccyx, the other on her heart (from the back), and place your lips on her lips or on her cheek or ear. An exchange of breath is an exchange of souls. Play together in a curious, tender, passionate, and creative way.

* Connect your breathing, yoni, heart, and third eye with those of your partner. Meanwhile, hold your partner's pelvis; you can massage or vibrate it. Play on her tender skin or her heaving flesh with all your desire. Take your time; be gentle, supportive, honest; and communicate with language as well.

* As your partner breathes out, you take in that energy, all the power that is flowing through your partner. So drink in the energy as you breathe in; feel how it swings back and forth between the two of you. Be patient when dealing with hindrances. Let your chakras bloom, and let the energy of free self-expression open your throat. Your pelvises rock like waves. Let the energy you have taken in flow all the way to your crown; imagine the path. You can change your position while rocking. Repeatedly draw the energy into your third eye and hold it there for a while.

* You can also lay your mouth on your partner's so that, through mouth contact and alternate breathing, you drink each other in and let yourself be drunk in by your partner. This can increase your feeling of melting together.

* Spacelessness and timelessness grow up out of the sexual energy that flows together between you. Once the river has passed the rapids, it can become a calm, wide stream that carries both of you. Hold the strength of your spirit in your third eye, lay your forehead on your partner's, and relax. This is the tantric kiss. Breathe your "self" out, deep and wide, and include your partner in your breathing space. Your soul flies all over, your spirit expands, your energy grows more and more delicate and fuses with your partner's. Feel how your spirit and soul are infinite in their freedom. Love, peace, wisdom—these states all develop through the unity of two lovers.

* Slowly open your eyes, attuned to this knowledge, and look into your partner's eyes: "I honor you as an aspect of my own self. I see

us as different but equally vibrating, connected embodiments of
_____ (fill in the blank; for example, the goddess
Tara)." Now slowly separate, and sit across from each other.

✳ Relax together by "spooning" or lying together in some way that is
comfortable for both of you.

✳ After this comes a long silence; a gentle, step-by-step separation
from each other; an exchange where you name your experiences but
do not try to analyze them, instead simply marveling at them.

CREATIVE WAYS TO DEAL WITH STUMBLING BLOCKS
For novices, the yab-yum position can easily grow uncomfortable. The alternate position, with one leg over and one leg under the other's (scissor position), is usually only temporarily easier. There's only one thing to do: *Practice!* Or try out different versions of melting-together bodies—on a chair, lying on top of each other, standing together, or lying on your sides.

VARIATIONS AND SUGGESTIONS
The pelvic rocking as well as the breathing in the yab-yum position can be either parallel or alternate—there is neither "right" nor "wrong" here, simply different sensations in different positions.

𝒲 Exercise 51: Sex-magical skills

Sexual magic is an integration and development of the previous games and exercises. It has to do with the art of using sexual energy, as the fastest and strongest type of energy we have, to build up a field where all our wishes, goals, and longings gain strength for their fulfillment. So we use the creative power of our laps and our ability to transform this energy in all directions to make visions materialize; that is, we concentrate this power's energy so much that it takes on outer forms as well as inner ones.

Magic is

✳ gaining creative power by being in harmony with the world

✳ being one with nature and its laws

✳ the playful dissolution of old borders and limitations

✳ a "double-edged sword": on one hand, a powerful influence toward healing and growth; on the other hand, the destruction of myself or the other

Sex magic is

✳ a delightful meditation that creates a big, wide space where I can plant the seed of my heart's desires and visions and let it grow

✳ an honest desire, benefitting my development, to give maximal power to satisfaction through sexual joys and their expansion

✳ the possibility to transform the powers that oppose my magical thinking and goal-oriented actions. This frees further strength for the manifestation of my visions

✳ in short, the most pleasurable way to work powerfully

GOAL

With sex magic, you can reach goals *that benefit you and do not harm others.* For example, you can grant visions reality; bring love into the world; and let yourself spread out, attaining healing for yourself and others as well as the wisdom of a sympathetic heart.

TIME AND EXTERNAL PREPARATIONS

About one or two hours. The exercise can be repeated many times with the same goal (up to twenty-one times, a number of repetitions that helps the experiences become a part of the subconscious, which helps them become habit more easily).

STEP BY STEP

Below are listed the steps, roughly in order, by which you access the magical creative power of sexual energy. Each step is made up of a series of activities, some of which have already been described in detail and which I will only mention briefly here.

✳ *Creating a safe room and a good emotional foundation with each other:* Cleansing yourself inside and out, clearing relationship difficulties out of the way, drawing a protective circle around your mutual pleasure space.

❊ *Fanning the sexual flames:* Sexual breathing, PC muscle contractions, pelvic rocking; self-love and responsibility for yourself; erotic massages.

❊ *Awakening the inner magician:* A fantasy journey to states of positive power, a creative trance-journey to the ideal inner beloved, fantastical self-arousal.

❊ *Removing inner hindrances:* Letting go of feelings, tuning in on the heart level, showing and healing wounds, the laughing belly.

❊ *Awakening your wild self:* Fire-breathing orgasm, meditation of the wild fire-woman, dance of the she-demons, groaning yoni.

❊ *Creating a magical vision:* Fantasy journeys (clear goals and visions of the healing, development, and cultivation of your own sexuality); drawing a picture to accompany them; finding a symbol; drawing a new picture with the symbol in the foreground and a simple, easy-to-remember composition.

❊ *Creating and charging a magical symbol:* Taking your partner as strengthener and mirror, chakra wave, chakra breathing (there is a CD with this same title for a chakra-breathing meditation; see the Resources section).

❊ *Creating maximal sexual pleasure:* "MMM," ESO, yab-yum.

❊ *Fusing orgasmic "high paths" with magic and with your symbol:* When bundling orgasmic energy (see "MMM," Exercise 48), intensely imagine the picture of the magic symbol; when distributing the energy, imagine that the symbol is flowing through all your body parts like new information.

❊ *Projection into the astral net:* "Releasing" the symbol through the seventh chakra, and imagining that the symbol is being breathed upward through the inner flute of the chakras, leaving the material body through the crown chakra, traveling through the aura, and spreading out more and more.

❊ *Checking the results:* Being awake to encounters and events, patient expectation, questions of interpretation.

CREATIVE WAYS TO DEAL WITH STUMBLING BLOCKS
Sometimes the goal is not stated clearly enough, or the symbol is not simplified enough. The result is often confusion in the process. Therefore, keep it short and sweet; simplicity is wisdom.

VARIATIONS AND SUGGESTIONS

* Your personal magic will be stronger the greater your sexual energy is.

* The creative energy of sexuality is in no way limited to the creation of children.

* Helpful qualities: patience, being tenacious and watchful, remaining goal-oriented *and* passive.

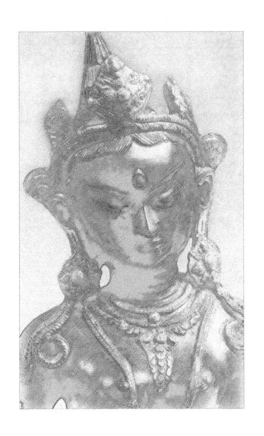

☙ CHAPTER 10 ☙

Pleasure as a Way of Meditation

*T*he following three meditations have one thing in common: They serve to pave the way to pure joy for you and your sexual energy, which perhaps has just been aroused in one of the sexual games and massages. When your energy is moving in that direction, a wide space of happiness, peace, and animated abundance can open up to you. It can spread with every breath you take, until it becomes one with the collective wide space in which fullness becomes emptiness and emptiness becomes fullness. The feeling of being protected in this wide space (for me and perhaps also for you) makes the meaning of life sensually palpable.

ℐ Exercise 52: Female visions of joy

The most important organ for the cultivation of love, pleasure, and passion is your heart. The following meditation is concerned with transformational processes and with the subtle energy that is developed by opening the heart chakra.

GOAL
Giving in to the quieter and more delicate movements, sounds, and emotions.

TIME AND EXTERNAL PREPARATIONS
At least an hour in a quiet, warm room. You can record the following instructions on a tape ahead of time so that you can give in completely to your feelings during the meditation.

STEP BY STEP

Phase 1: Light fountain (standing, fifteen minutes)
With your tongue on the roof of your mouth, audibly draw in air through your open mouth until your lungs are completely full. Then breathe out completely, with a long "Haaah." As you breathe in, draw your hands up over your head with outstretched arms; as you breathe out, bring them down along your sides. Imagine that white or pastel light is flowing through your whole body as you breathe in, filling you completely, and flowing down the sides of your body as you breathe out. This closes the circle of light. (If you are familiar with breathing and movement, you can

experiment with slowly increasing the length of the pauses between breaths in and out.)

Phase 2: Song of the heart (standing, fifteen minutes)
Now imagine that your heart is being filled with delightful warmth with every breath you take in. Your whole heart region grows larger and larger until it finally includes the rest of your body. Accompanied by soft music, let your heart become a musical instrument; let it vibrate, shake, and ring. Find within yourself more and more of your heart's song. Open yourself with your voice for your inner sounds and noises, and let your hands and arms, as well as your whole body, move with the song. You can let words and sentences come spontaneously, or express yourself in an imaginary language. Give in to the experience completely and *become* singing!

Phase 3: Giving in to the light (sitting up straight, fifteen minutes)
Sit up on your knees (another straight-backed position would work as well), and stretch your arms upward. Wait, using soft breathing, until you feel full of heart-warmth. Then draw your hands to your heart center, and from there go into a forward bend. Let your forehead and palms rest on the floor until you are completely empty again.

Repeat this process using your own rhythm.

Phase 4: Silence (sitting or lying on your back, fifteen minutes)
Now you can decide whether you want to be in a sitting or a lying down position. Close your eyes. Let yourself sink into calmness, but remain as awake as possible. Observe everything that enters your field of perception. After about fifteen minutes, stretch your body out well and observe yourself with tenderness and loving attention from within.

Below are some ideas for words that you might want to say or to have said to you during each phase. Here, too, remember to use only what truly works for you; invent your own words if you like.

Light fountain

My breathing opens up, broad and deep, and through it I open myself to light and joy. With every breath, light flows through my body, flows all the way through me and far beyond me. I open myself up, make myself broad for the light's circulation. With every breath, I take in the whole of pleasurable life; it flows into me and fills me more and more. I am connected to a gently bubbling source of the rivers of female energy, a part of the divine female power that fills me more and more. I open the borders of my fear, and women's power from different times and places pours, flows, breathes, and becomes a part of me. The fullness of various women's lives fills my consciousness, and in the name of this fullness I greet this hour and everything that is now a part of me and my life. I relax into the fullness of being and am open to love, freedom, and joy. I am now connected to the great circulatory system of female power and to the female love present in the whole world—a love for women that leads me, carries me, and accompanies me in life.

I feel a new strength within me, and I know that it is the strength that flows from the source of my deepest female strength, namely the desire in my lap that leaves me completely infused and fulfilled.

With each new breath, I give myself away; I share my being with life and with women (or with this one woman who is here with me), and I am continually filled anew. The more I give and share, the more this giving and sharing flows back to me.

In greater and stronger waves, light, pleasure, and joy flow through my being. And with this opening, in this letting go, in this *yes,* a powerful and tender love energy comes to me from everywhere. It touches me gently and powerfully. It touches the slumbering love and joy within me.

I become more and more a channel of light, a source of pleasure, and a vessel of joy that overflows and fills everything that is within my consciousness. I am light and love. I am joy and satisfaction. I am unity. All the pleasure of living, all the pleasure of womanhood to which I have opened myself, flows and bubbles up within me, laughs and sings with me.

I am a woman, connected to the pleasure and power and fullness of many generations of women who together embody female goddesses.

Song of the heart

From my inner satisfaction, I find my tone. My body begins to sway gently, and I grant my voice free expression. The fullness of my heart flows into my song. I let myself be filled by my song, and I become more and more a joyful expression of my heart.

Because of the overflowing joy within me, my movements and my voice grow more and more powerful. I let my joy, my love, my longing, everything that is within me, sing through me. I let my female soul be expressed through my song. I let my being sing through me, and I connect myself with everything that exists. I sing the song of my heart, the song of my joy, the song of my love, the song of my power as a woman, the song of my truth, the song of my devotion.

The song of my heart becomes a gift to the world of women. I recognize the gift I have received that allows me to participate and share in female divinity. Everything in me begins to sing, and everything around me joins in. With the song of my heart, I connect myself to the light of totality.

Giving in to the light

In devotion to the moment, I open myself to the light. Generously, I pass this light on to the earth, to life. Devotion occurs in the letting go of fear, in the letting go of my boundaries, in the love of totality.

The light of joy fills my inner world, fills my whole life, my being. I am now ready to feel my love within me and to distribute it. I let myself grow still, come home to myself, in the connection of joy and light. I let myself feel how, in this moment, I am one with the light of divine female energy.

CREATIVE WAYS TO DEAL WITH STUMBLING BLOCKS

If, despite all these incitements to joy, you feel more anger or sadness, allow yourself to have those feelings and their corresponding sounds, and play with them inwardly, trying to use and transform their energy. For example, you might transform the energy into joyful, survival-oriented rage or into that small sense of melancholy that can accompany deep, quiet joy.

🐚 Exercise 53: Full-moon meditation

This is a meditation developed to train for ecstasy and love. It connects all tantrikas—that is, all the people who concern themselves with the meaning and practice of tantra and who do the meditation quietly, either alone or with others, every Sunday afternoon at 2:00 P.M. Pacific time.

GOAL

The subtle energetic connection of all tantrikas beyond geographical and temporal separation.

TIME AND EXTERNAL PREPARATIONS

About twenty to thirty minutes. As preparation, imagine all the people you personally associate with the concept of tantra or love-pleasure.

STEP BY STEP

* Breathe into your heart with slow, deep, gentle breaths, broadening your heart chakra. Then open both hands, with your left palm facing up and your right palm facing down, and imagine that the left palm is opened for a loving touch from other tantrikas; you draw the energy of this touch into your heart as you breathe in, and as you breathe out, you let it flow through your right hand to other tantrikas. In this way, you create a balanced flow of energy through your body (maybe you can feel the energy flow in your palms?), and you close the energy circuit with all other real and imagined beings.

* Now create a vertical energy flow by breathing through the inner flute of the chakras and by pausing after each breath drawn up to the crown chakra until the breath comes out by itself. After breathing out to the root chakra, pause again until your breath comes in by itself. In your imagination, let roots grow out of your kundalini point at the coccyx or out of your yoni. As you breathe in, draw warm, nourishing energy from these roots, and imagine a plant growing upward along your spine, all the way up to your crown.

* Imagine a star in the sky (if it is evening or night where you are, you might even pick out a nice, big one), and feel the rays it emits. A clear, bright ray hits your crown and fills you up.

* Feel the horizontal and the vertical as they connect in your heart. Send your breath through your heart and awaken it so that it can

bloom and grow larger. Coax out the healing, melting energy that now spreads through your body into every cell.

✳ Light flows into every pore, light through which your energy field shines with all the colors of the rainbow, growing larger. It creates a delicate, thin bubble around you. Slowly let it grow larger, encompassing your partner or your surroundings with glowing, colorful light. Your colorful energy bubble then goes out beyond the walls to include the house, the neighborhood, the country, the continent, the whole blue planet.

✳ Send your energy into the waters—the rivers, seas, and oceans. Imagine a clear freshness and let it become even purer. Then send your love into the air so that balance is restored to the atmosphere. And send healing love to the plants—their roots, stems, and leaves—so that they can transform the light into joy and good health. And send love and healing to the animals so that they might eat the plants and have their habitat preserved, and might live in the joy of being.

✳ And send your love to all women. Feel your sympathy for all women, for their worries and hurts. For a moment, picture yourself being connected with all women in love and joy. Send your love to the hearts you especially like. Surround them with your love, your understanding, and your sympathy.

✳ Then take back your freely flowing energy, a little at a time, with each breath—back into the room. Now the environment includes only your partner. Let the energy bubble grow smaller until it is just a glow around you. Let it grow even smaller, all the way into your heart. Feel the strength to heal, to love, to sympathize, and to understand others in the middle of your heart. Then take your right hand and lay it on your heart. Add your left hand to it. Continue breathing into the center.

✳ Whisper, "Yes, I love myself." Listen to your heart. Feel it and know that the strength to love yourself gives you the strength to love others. Love the others as you love yourself. Slowly come back to the room. Be completely there and awake, and open your eyes.

CREATIVE WAYS TO DEAL WITH STUMBLING BLOCKS
You may think you should see your energy as healing love for all living things. However, this is not about over- or underestimating your powers, but rather about seeing yourself as a droplet of water in the ocean.

VARIATIONS AND SUGGESTIONS
Originally, of course, this meditation was meant for both men and women; I have used only the female version in order to emphasize the connection of women to one another. You can vary this aspect of the meditation if you like.

Exercise 54: Meditation on love for yourself
(Adapted from Jeru Kabbal's breathing meditation for women.)

Love for yourself begins with and lives through conscious breathing. If we understand conscious, deepened, and expanded breathing as one of the keys to conscious, deepened, and expanded desire, it makes sense to deepen and stretch out *all* pleasurable experiences through breathing.

GOAL
Integrating past experiences—pleasurable as well as painful—through breathing, and practicing enjoying the present moment without clinging to it.

TIME AND EXTERNAL PREPARATIONS
At least forty-five to sixty minutes; but you might leave yourself a little more time to become still. For this meditation it's very important that you be in a room where you can make all kinds of emotional sounds. The instructions contain several repetitions that help you concentrate your spirit on your breathing over and over again, and that help lead you away from intellectual analysis back to a real perception of the moment. If you like, record the instructions on a cassette tape so that you can completely submit to the workings of your inner process.

    If you have a partner who is not participating, you can ask that person to gently support your stomach breathing by laying a hand on your belly.

It is important that you decide how long you would like to have this support and how strong it should be.

As musical support, you can use any kind of music that lets you sway gently, touches your heart, and lasts at least forty-five minutes. If you like classical music, here are a few examples that can support the different breath frequencies and are easy to find, so that you can put together your own collection: "Baccarole" (Offenbach); "Air" (Bach); "Ritual Fire Dance" (M. de Falla); "From Holberg's Time" (Grieg); "Morning Mood" (Massenet); "Angelic Touch" (Seiler); "Genesis" (Sandelan).

STEP BY STEP

* Lie down or sit in a comfortable position. Your clothing should be loose and comfortable and your stomach relaxed; otherwise it will be hard to breathe deeply. Allow your belly to relax more and more; once you're concentrating on it, breathe completely into your belly so that it pushes outward. Then keep breathing in until your lungs are completely full, too.

* It's a good idea to exert yourself a little at the beginning; that is, to consciously draw the air into your lungs. You can breathe through your nose or your mouth—the main thing is to take in oxygen. Each breath should be full and deep. (If you are accustomed to shallow breathing, it might be hard for you to significantly increase the volume of your breath in your stomach area. If this is the case, it may help to imagine that you are an accordion, for example, stretching out and making emotive sounds, gradually collapsing again, and then stretching out anew.)

* Observe your thoughts. It's natural to have thoughts, but be aware that you are not *made up of* these thoughts. You don't need to spend any energy on these thoughts.

* Concentrate completely on your breathing. You are taking in more oxygen than your body needs, and thereby you are building up your energy. You keep coming back to your breathing; you put all your intelligence, all your attention, all your energy into breathing. You keep breathing into your relaxed belly, and then you try to stretch out your lungs completely. It is normal for thoughts to be

present. They are the product of your reason—you do not need to obey them or fight them. Just don't give them any energy. Your energy is going to your breathing. You are building up your energy. You will then trust in this energy—it's your energy, and you know you can trust it.

* No matter what you are thinking or feeling, keep coming back to your breathing. Breathe fully and deeply, fully and deeply.

* You breathe into your relaxed belly, filling your lungs completely with every breath. Every breath is important. Every breath brings life, new vitality, new energy that rinses you; every breath cleanses you, expands your power, and finally transforms you. Breathe in deeply and fully. Always come back to your breathing.

* If new thoughts surface, let them come and then go; tell yourself that you do not have to follow these thoughts. You also don't need to fight with them. You can simply leave them there and concentrate on your breathing. You will build up your energy through your breathing. The deeper and more fully you breathe in, the stronger your experience will be. Breathe deeply and fully. Even if you have unfamiliar physical sensations, allow them; accept them and continue breathing. It may be that memories or emotions come up later. Allow these to happen too, and accept them. However, be sure to concentrate on your breathing.

* You are building up your energy. With every breath, you expand your energy field. With every breath, you strengthen your energy field. It may be that you feel like you need to laugh or cry or scream. Allow and accept these feelings, but don't give them any energy. You are giving all your energy to your breathing. You are not suppressing these feelings. You are simply not giving them any energy. With every breath, you open yourself up to life. You breathe your own life in with every breath. Always come back to your breathing, continuing to build up your energy.

* You breathe deeply into your relaxed belly. Each breath brings new life, vitality, good health. Each breath cleanses you. Each breath

expands your energy field. You breathe your own life in with each breath. You open yourself wider and wider, breathing fully and deeply.

✳ Drink in, breathe in life. Let yourself expand. Allow everything, accept everything. Drink in life, breathe in life. Breathe fully into your lungs. Open yourself wider. Fill your lungs with air, with life. Keep breathing. Allow everything, accept everything. Keep coming back to your breathing. Breathe deeply and fully.

✳ Allow everything, accept everything, but always keep coming back to the breathing, and stay conscious of the process. You are building up your energy, so you are breathing very strongly now. And you now breathe as quickly and as strongly and as fully as you possibly can. Breathe very powerfully, allowing everything, accepting everything. Breathe powerfully. Breathe fully and deeply. Relax the belly completely. Relax the belly.

✳ Keep concentrating on your breathing, avoiding any other thoughts. Feel yourself filling with power, with energy, with life. Feel the miracle that you are, and intensify this power with every breath. Enjoy your power, your strength, your ability to concentrate on your breathing. Open yourself up and breathe. Enjoy life; breathe and open yourself. Keep breathing.

✳ Now breathe very slowly. Breathe fully and deeply again. You are breathing into a relaxed belly.

✳ Now imagine that you are sitting in front of a sunrise; the sky grows lighter and lighter, and the sun comes up over the horizon. Feel this energy, this new awakening, this new beginning. Breathe the streaming sunlight in. Breathe slowly, fully, and deeply. Open yourself. Keep breathing fully and deeply.

✳ Continue to concentrate on your breathing—not on the music, not on any outside sounds. These are allowed to be there but should stay somewhere on the edge of your consciousness. The most important thing is your breathing. Keep breathing, breathing in life fully and deeply. Open yourself to this moment. Feel the sun, higher now in the sky, very warm and friendly. You breathe in this warmth, you breathe in this light. Keep breathing, concentrating on the breathing. Keep breathing fully and deeply.

✳ Keep breathing, keep breathing. You are breathing deeply into your belly.

✳ Now breathe more into your heart region. Let your heart open up to your life, to you yourself. Open your heart to yourself. And keep breathing, allowing all feelings, and keep coming back to the breathing. Concentrate on your continued breathing.

✳ Don't get involved in your emotions. Allow and accept them, and come back to the breathing. Don't give the emotions any energy. Keep breathing. Now breathe a little more slowly, gently, softly. But always keep breathing and concentrating on the breathing.

✳ Now allow yourself to feel the beautiful, delicate aspects of yourself—those delicate qualities that you have but very often forget about. Feel how the music mirrors this part of you. Keep breathing. Accept the old behavioral patterns, the old value judgments, the feelings from the basement of your past that may yet come up; allow them, but do not give them any energy.

✳ Stay concentrated on your breathing. The breathing is now, the breathing is being in the present, is the truth of your being. Your thoughts come from the past, which is long gone. Those old patterns are completely harmless if you remain in the present. You can free yourself from the old patterns simply by not giving them any energy and not fighting them; instead, you concentrate on the present, on your breathing.

✳ You have refreshed your body, you have renewed your soul; you have let many things go from your subconscious, even if you don't know exactly what they were. You feel completely new, completely awake, somehow lighter and cleaner. You may have the feeling that you are more present, that you are more *here*, that the real, true you is here. And if you have let go of the old patterns, you feel smarter, wiser, more loving. You can use this time to speak with yourself, to give yourself advice, to support yourself, since you are so clear right now.

✳ Imagine that a great rose-colored light is emanating from your heart. This rose-colored light grows stronger and stronger until your whole body is enveloped in the light. Let yourself be embraced, caressed, supported by this light. Allow yourself to love yourself. You have so much love to give. You often give so little to yourself. Let this great light nourish you, support you, warm you. And think about what a beautiful woman you are when you are full of desire. And imagine that you are watching out for yourself, taking care of yourself. Remind yourself that you are now a strong, adult woman. In this moment you can let all the old patterns fall, so let go of them. You are no longer the baby, the child, the girl that you once were. All the old strategies don't count anymore; you don't need them anymore. Now you can live in freedom, observing each moment by itself. And trust yourself in the present. And for a moment, now, imagine your life the way you'd like it to be and the way it could look. And with your inner eye, see yourself in your life. See how open, how strong, how beautiful you are. Today you will have the opportunity to come a step closer to this image. You simply need to recognize the opportunity to do so: the opportunity to not give in to the old habits, the opportunity to take this new path. Have the courage to try out something new, to find a new way, and look forward to the unknown. Feel it out once more; look inside to see if there is anything else you want to say to yourself.

✳ Then let yourself grow very still, ready to receive the flow of life.

✳ Remain seated as long as you want. When you are ready, stand up and go.

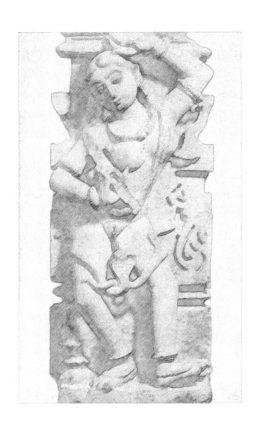

➤ CHAPTER II ☞

Concluding Without Ending

233

*L*ove lives through loving human beings. If love were a separate being, it would best express itself through sex, over and over again, and through the most varied forms of sex. It would want to spread in all directions and land back in our soul's body as an extended and refined spiritual force, to revive it, and to gently strengthen the connection to our love partners.

For me, this *integration of sex and spirituality* is one of the most important steps we women can take in a world of separation, alienation, and devaluation of both life forces, steps that are so necessary to preserving our world.

All the practical instructions offered in this book serve to awaken, cultivate, and expand our sexual energy in the widest sense. The more sexual our spirituality becomes, the more pleasurable and "closer to earth" our flights to spiritual heights will be. And the more spiritual our sexuality becomes, the more expanded and refined every sexual vibration will be. To me, both taken together comprise the wild-tender expression of female power, which, instead of oppressing others, becomes only possible in a respectful, lively encounter with myself and others. Such lust-power (instead of the usual lust for power) can have a healing effect far beyond our individual pleasure.

Here's my down-to-earth, optimistic conclusion: Affecting the world in a healing way can be pure pleasure, and sexual pleasure is the easiest and at the same time most powerful way of radiating joyful energy into the world.

So have fun playing, practicing, and feeling, however and wherever your spiritual-sexual energy carries you!

Appendixes

An end to the topic of sex is indeed not in sight. Instead, here are two appendixes that could by themselves make two separate books, as the topics they address open up special spaces for our sexual force: "Lesbian Love as a Form of Self-Love" (Appendix A) and "Sexual Energy as a Healing Force" (Appendix B).

Let yourself be inspired where you become curious and draw boundaries where you feel aversion. In any case, allow yourself again and again to create new forms and rooms for your sexual-spiritual energy and to share them with others with courage and pleasure!

APPENDIX A

Lesbian Love as a Form of Self-Love

*L*esbian love means encountering your own (sexual) self in the mirror of similarity. This means a *compounded increase of female qualities,* including biographical and actual roles, feelings, strengths and weaknesses. Such a state of affairs creates a high emotional density that can intensify any existing feelings—either in the direction of love, passion, tenderness, happiness, peace, and security, or in the direction of hate, aggression, fear, or pain. In order to keep this high intensity from becoming an internal and external sensory overload, it is necessary to draw clear boundaries and to switch back and forth between experiences of blissful fusion and practices that distance you from your partner and raise your self-awareness. All this makes it necessary to reintegrate those so-called "male aspects" of your being—qualities that women generally project onto men—into the relationship, either on your own or as a division of labor. These qualities are crucial for your own vitality, for your own integrity, and for creatively shaping your sexual relationship (e.g., active seduction, or taking the initiative to make the next move).

Despite all the steps that have been made toward tolerance, lesbian women must still deal with discrimination, open or subtle prejudices, "pathologization," and the like—and not only from the outside, but also from other lesbians as well as from their own subconscious voices. This is compounded by an extremely subtle form of oppression: In many official arenas, the lesbian lifestyle is either not mentioned at all or is not recognized as an equal way of living. A crazy situation ensues: Your own personally experienced reality seems unreal, since it cannot be seen or named in the collective (and therefore reality-constructing) mirror. This makes lesbian networks, coming-out announcements for the general public, political discussions, and other public discussions of women's sexual wishes, boundaries, norms, and longings all the more important. Also important is having an enjoyable sexual life—at the very least in your own bedroom—while putting a stop to your internalized prejudices and negative ideas. The fact that lesbians define their identities not solely but *also* through their sexuality and the fact that lesbian couples rarely receive societal recognition both give *sexuality as an identity-creating moment and as a magical place of confirmation and strengthening in a romantic relationship* a high priority in everyday life, with the result that disruptions in this area can easily become threats to relationships and identities.

In a misogynistic, homophobic society like ours, women loving women is a special art that requires specific capabilities and skills. These are not necessarily given to us, but we can gradually cultivate them. They include

* love for yourself as a woman; desiring yourself on a physical, metaphysical, intellectual, and spiritual level

* the ability to fall in love with similarity rather than exclusively with difference

* the ability to increase sexual arousal without the impulse of gender tension

* flexibility in moving between intimacy and distance, as well as the symbiosis and difference of individuals

* openness to creating more intimacy—for example, by getting rid of your fear of closeness and your tendency toward "mother-transference" (i.e., emotionally confusing the roles of your mother and your current lover)

* activity/initiative and devotion/*affidamento* (in the sense of the Italian women's movement: trusting yourself to another with her particular skills and possibilities)

* creative use in assigning roles without the security of norms, rules, and role models

* a self-aware drawing of as well as the courageous broadening of boundaries

* the ability to deal confidently with both open and subtle discrimination;

* differentiated strategies for coming out in various political and social contexts

* dealing with the misogyny and homophobia in your own feminist subconscious

* the development and practice of ways of speaking and thinking that provide room for female contexts and relationships

* the ability to orient yourself and move in very different social and normative worlds

* building networks and support structures in which your own relationships can be embedded and which can help stabilize them

* a conscious decision to grow out of the passive victim role, and a conscious use and encouragement of your own capabilities and talents in the art of women's love

Realities of Lesbian Relationships

The following relationship qualities and tendencies often develop as foundations for sexual encounters between women:

LESBIAN RELATIONSHIPS PREFER TO BLOOM IN PRIVATE
SPACES AND NEED SECURE BORDERS TO THE OUTSIDE.

When we consider that there is little collective confirmation of lesbian relationships and that confirmation through the subculture of other lesbian networks is underdeveloped and often even ambivalent (due to differing values, jealousy, envy, and competition), it makes sense that there seems to be more fear (e.g., of rejection) in collective areas, along with an increased need for protection in most lesbian relationships than in most heterosexual relationships. In addition, women have learned for centuries to see the public sphere as men's terrain and the private sphere as that of women. In terms of emotions, the slogans of the new women's movement, such as "the private is political," have made little difference. In a social atmosphere where lesbians are at best tolerated or marketed as exotic, where lesbian love is not automatically considered to be a normal variant, only privacy and select islands of separatism offer a little protection and safety—even if we still can't escape the patriarchal thought patterns in our own heads.

To me, the brilliant thing about lesbian play-parties or sexual playshops (places to play within the framework of seminars, workshops, etc.) is that they can help you build the courage to open up your own space of intimacy in the presence of several women, which then rewards you with a tremendous increase of your own lustful energy.

LESBIAN RELATIONSHIPS LIVE MORE FROM THE REFLECTION OF SIMILARITY THAN FROM DIFFERENCE.

This can encourage the well-known leaning toward symbiosis and can expand into unselfconscious devotion or even self-destruction. Since, for many lesbians, acknowledging differences and distance seems like a threat to the relationship, they often reject the paths to individuation that their relationships—and they as individuals—need for further development. Frequently, roles are divided up within a couple: One person emphasizes the difference and distance, the other the similarity and closeness. The one who emphasizes distance is often the one who wins out.

On the other hand, the mirroring of similarities (for example, in female identities, life stories, physicalities, methods of communication) means a greater amount of closeness, intimacy, and blurring of borders. This can translate into greater pleasure in sexual fusion. However, it can also call up early mother-memories from the symbiotic phase (i.e., a "transference" of old roles, feelings, and behaviors from a young girl's experience with her mother or the first important person in her life), causing a great deal of pain stemming from early and current deficiencies and disturbances. As a result, there is particular pressure to get rid of or at least to lessen the old childhood roles (e.g., the hungry and needy child who insists on her right to nourishment and affection). This can be done, for instance, by giving the adult woman enough hugs so that the drive to fall into her beloved's arms the minute she walks through the door (regardless of whether there are eggs in the grocery bags) is somewhat lessened. If a woman does not take active responsibility for her childish need to catch up, it will be difficult for her to react as an adult (either sexually or communicatively) in an intimate relationship with another woman. Her old childhood needs will push themselves into the foreground sooner than she or her partner would like. If this is not possible for the individual, the energy of old patterns of disturbance (for example, aggressive insistence on the childish satisfaction of needs or frustrated rage when her partner refuses to take on the nurturing mother role) can easily become an explosive volcanic energy that is expressed through violence, blind destructive rage, a cold shoulder, or abrupt separation strategies.

THE MAJORITY OF LESBIAN RELATIONSHIPS ARE INFLUENCED BY PLENTY OF COMMUNICATION, CLOSENESS, AND THE ATTEMPT, EVEN IN AN ARGUMENT, TO GIVE HIGHER STATUS TO THE RELATIONSHIP THAN TO SELF-ASSERTION.

Here we see how much lesbian relationships are influenced by the increased use of female negotiation strategies, since most women learn at an early age not only to value human relationships, but also to make sacrifices for them (sacrificing, for example, the furthering of their own interests) and to define themselves by their relationships. This behavior, too, has its own consequences. On the one hand, arguments become less hierarchical, being principally between equals; thus, more constructive strategies are chosen. On the other hand, the personal sacrifices made for the common good, for harmony in the relationship, are often so great that each woman's own path, her individuality, falls by the wayside; this can silently poison the vitality of the relationship (for example, in the form of unexpressed resentment). Couples can become more and more alike on the outside as a result of all this striving for harmony, while inside they are not even able to vegetate in a state of pleasant boredom alongside one another without feeling frustrated, knowing that expressing individual sexual desires or addressing conflicts of interest is seen as a dangerous step in the direction of breaking up.

LESBIAN RELATIONSHIPS TEND TO BE MARKED BY A HIGH LEVEL OF FEMALE CARING FOR ONE ANOTHER—OR BY THE OPPOSITE, DEMONSTRATIVELY SHOWN.

Here, too, it becomes clear how much female socialization affects current lesbian relationships. Caring, sympathy, helpfulness, responsibility, caution, and maternal attention are traditional forms of female ways of loving, seen in lesbian relationships either in an emphasized form or in aversion. This means that either there is, from one or both sides, a great deal of caring and nurturing in the relationship, or the rejection of traditional women's roles creates an often stubborn-seeming defensiveness against any kind of caring. Sometimes the result is that an attitude like "Every woman for herself" is taken to extremes, and often the care for what is common, for the relationship, falls away.

LESBIAN RELATIONSHIPS OFTEN DEVELOP QUICKLY, FROM A HIGH LEVEL OF NEED.

When there is a great need for closeness and connection (sometimes even dependency), the first phase of being in love is not followed by any clear phase analogous to an "engagement." One or both parties is already talking about a committed relationship without reaching a rational, well-founded understanding about entering a commitment with all of its requirements (e.g., the idea of spending a lengthy period of your life with this person). The results may range from a sudden breakup after the first few arguments, to the development of unconscious structures of dependency without reaching clear and responsible agreements (e.g., about dividing up roles or about differing interests). The common things about these dependencies are not just feelings of helplessness and loss of autonomy (which add up to a loss of pride and self-awareness), but also, after a while, even the development of hatred. Since these feelings particularly cannot be expressed in a situation of mutual dependence, it rots away as an excess of energy in the internal organs. Finally, it becomes a poisonous mixture that can either lead to sudden aggressive outbursts or can slowly draw the woman or women into common suffering, like a creeping nerve gas that can make the skin insensitive or painfully oversensitive, cause eczema, or block the fine energy flow of desire at any number of points.

IN LESBIAN RELATIONSHIPS, MANY CONFLICTS ARISE IN SYN-CHRONIZING DIFFERENT SCHEDULES.

As a rule, lesbians must support themselves. This means that both partners are usually working (or looking for work) and have to take care of a household "on the side." And more and more often, there are children as well. It is a feature of our time that people's schedules (work schedules, time for relaxing, time for concentrating exclusively on the relationship) are quite full—and time always seems to be too short anyway. To this is added the fact that both partners usually place a high value on "relationship care," which means that the private time that is left often comes into conflict with your individual wishes and the demands of your social circle (friends, work colleagues), desires and needs that cannot be fulfilled during relationship time. In sexual togetherness, too, rhythms (of arousal and orgasms) are more different than is commonly recognized. So women—even with all their similarities and their inclination to merge with one another—must make arrangements that value and sometimes deny each others' differences. If they can also let go of the norm of regular mutual orgasms, they can come together in wild-tender arousal or in calm fusion, even if they don't come at the same time.

LESBIAN RELATIONSHIPS CAN BE OVERSHADOWED BY THE COMPOUNDED EFFECTS OF VIOLENCE AND ABUSE.

When two women enter into a romantic relationship together, the probability that one or both have been the victim of sexual violence and other forms of male violence, either as a child or as an adult, is doubled. This means that many of the effects of violence can cause massive damage to their relationship (through a lack of trust, learned helplessness, and other victim identities). On the other hand, a relationship built fundamentally on trust can provide the space needed to grow beyond past hurtful experiences. Still, the ability to be insightful is often undercut by an unconscious confusion of the new partner with earlier perpetrators, as well as the confusion of intimacy with pushing boundaries; thus, the partner must have a good sense of her own vulnerability in order to remain patient and supportive here. When both women are survivors of sexual violence, we can only imagine the complexity involved in maintaining useful and enjoyable communication between partners.

IN LESBIAN RELATIONSHIPS, SEXUAL SATISFACTION RISES AND FALLS WITH THE QUALITY OF THE EMOTIONAL RELATIONSHIP.

The reason for this is that many women see sex only in the context of amorousness, affairs, and romantic relationships, and these women value harmony, continuity, and frequent togetherness more than, say, their own desire. Another reason is the emphasis in society on sexual tension being created by gender differences. When we assume, though, that the fusion experienced in sex carries enormous power and stabilizing potential for the individual as well as for the relationship, it's really a shame to experience this potential only when everything else is going well.

I am not recommending alienated physical sex without emotional connection. I simply think that it is possible to create spaces (including timespaces) in every relationship where loving sexual encounters can occur, even if a fight hasn't been fought to the end yet or power struggles are occurring on other levels. (In other words, why do we allow problems in the relationship to affect our mutual sexuality, yet don't admit that our mutual sexuality has the power to affect or resolve the relationship problems?) Creating such a space requires an ability to move freely between desire and lack of desire and to consciously give your (mutual) desire more space. Sometimes a certain amount of *discipline* helps us cut off our preoccupation with fighting (or with lack of desire, pain, fear, or pressure to perform), both at a certain time and emotionally—in the same way that we are able to finish sex punctually in order to get to work. Of course, this is only possible with small to medium-sized arguments. In the case of discussions about breaking up or other things of that nature, it is probably better to focus your energy on the conflict. Unfortunately, in these cases the sexual encounter takes a hike too.

"Sex with your ex" usually builds on the illusion of a good breakup and the possibility of a new contact, free from old relationship patterns. This is where this type of situation often fails, too, because it ignores the deeper needs of one or both women. In the cases I know where women had wonderful sex with their exes, the relationship was usually far behind them. Both partners had put a lot of energy into a careful and unanimous separation, and they were not using one another to drive away their loneliness or as a defense against the fear of becoming involved in new relationships.

LONG-TERM LESBIAN RELATIONSHIPS, BY THEIR COMBINATION OF INTIMACY AND AUTONOMY, CAN OFFER PERSONAL ROOM FOR DEVELOPMENT TO ANYONE WHO CAN INTENSIVELY ENCOURAGE THE CREATION OF HER ADULT IDENTITY.

The following are some of the requirements for being involved with your sexuality, even in a long-term relationship:

* After the first phase of falling in love, you do not enter immediately into a tight bond; you give yourself time to create the relationship—time for a well-founded understanding to grow.

* There is room for the individual, that is, each has her own radius of action, and there are more or less clearly defined boundaries between the two individuals.

* There is room for intimacy (sexuality, security, trust-filled togetherness).

* There is time for one another, support on a daily basis, and realistic expectations of one another.

* There is a similar rhythm (at least time-wise) of symbiosis/fusion and individuation/definition.

* There is individual and mutual management of stressors and disturbances (work, performance pressure, other relationships, addictions, etc.).

✳ There is a willingness on both sides to out yourselves as a couple (of course, not everywhere or at all times) and to defend the borders of your "couple space" against attacks from the outside.

✳ Sexuality is used as a ritual place of power; not just during so-called vacations and celebrations, but also in everyday life (or everyday nights).

✳ There are flexible as well as fixed roles and divisions of labor in which an antihierarchical relationship with one another is emphasized, despite any concentration of forces in one area or another.

✳ There is a basic ability to fight and have conflicts. Fights are carried out *to their conclusion* (with breaks, if necessary), and serious excuses are accepted. This includes the willingness to let go of old injuries and to create (mutual) forms of repentance and reconciliation so that both can let go of their old feelings.

✳ It is made clear in words and actions that the other is treated with love and respect, and that differences are valued.

✳ There are transitional and renewal rituals (e.g., vacations, new mutual friends, new common activities) as well as a mutual openness toward new impulses regarding the relationship. Playing together and spending celebrations and holidays together is particularly emphasized.

✳ There is a need for constant growth and constant searching, both individually and as a couple.

✳ There is a fundamental willingness to acknowledge personal responsibility and to work on it (for example, if a woman needs to get rid of the maternal projections mentioned earlier, she must give herself what her childish side still needs rather than forcing her beloved into that role and then needing her terribly).

✳ Beyond neurotic feelings of guilt, there is a basic willingness to be found responsible or guilty in the egalitarian sense; that is, each person is responsible not only for her own well-being, but also for taking care of the relationship—through regular periods of cuddling, for example.

* Deficits in relationship skills or in managing everyday life are taken care of with communication, humor, and practice.

* "Yes" does not always automatically lose out against "no" but is always tested. For example, if one person wants sex now and the other does not, the naysayer does not automatically win; through an active understanding and consideration of the *no*, there are still possibilities: the art of sensitive and playful seduction on the part of the yes-sayer, for example, or the naysayer's trust that her appetite may emerge when she starts to eat....

* Simultaneously, both women develop such clear self-definitions that differences do not have to disappear in the quest for harmony; a consensus about difference and dissent is possible.

* Support networks and friends are sought out if the relationship requires outside help.

I see this list of requirements as neither binding nor even, in its ideal form, realizable. However, I believe they can improve the quality of sexual relationships and help make them more conscientious.

Sexual Energy as a Healing Force

$\mathcal{N}$ either active nor passive sexuality can magically cure illnesses or handicaps, but in certain phases of the healing process or the process of self-acceptance, sexuality can make room for the healing flow of energy; help transform energy; and promote vitality, physical sensations, and feelings of self-worth (through the empowering force of being recognized or the euphoric effect of endorphin release). These effects can greatly improve your subjective quality of life, which in turn is good for the healing process (e.g., by increasing immune defenses through feelings of joy and by improving oxygen intake with yelping, panting, and cheering).

But how is sexual healing supposed to work? Aren't illnesses associated with suffering, fear, and sadness? Sexual healing certainly doesn't work by denying these aspects; instead, it works through the attempt to open yourself cautiously to desire during respites from pain. The following is a short list of successfully tested, solid healing methods for playing with or encouraging your awakened sexual energy:

* SUGGESTIONS FOR SEXUAL HEALING

Theme	What to do	Effects on the healing processes
Fever	During a feverish state, consciously engage in erotic/sexual fantasies, visions, or daydreams.	Energizing effects for weakened states; dreams and visions about the healing process result in striving to reach it
Smiling inside	From the third eye, via the heart region, pour your inner smile into the sick organ; with each breath, imagine "waste matter" and pain being carried to the heart, where they are lovingly and smilingly revived. As a result, they can be transformed into warmth or accepting consciousness.	Comfortably relaxing into your pain; the feeling that all your pleasure organs have been enlarged
Sex in white	Engage, either actually or in your imagination, in sexual activities of all kinds in the starched white sheets of a hospital bed, with the thought that visitors might come at any time—or even the Catholic head nurse, who would find the intimate visit unhygienic as well!	Fun; improves circulation and encourages creativity; the allure of the forbidden; expands your previous sickness-related perceptions of the bed; creates joy and satisfaction
Silent enjoyment	For extreme weakness and resistance to touch, look at sexually attractive or seductive people or pictures.	Causes sorrow and pain over the life that cannot be fully enjoyed right now, but also creates a longing for it that encourages the healing process
Gentlest temptation	Especially for infections or moderate states of pain: Ignite and strengthen sexual energy by touching, petting, or gently kissing nonpainful areas, which steers awareness in their direction.	Pain is lessened, and the brain is confused by these conflicting sensations; you are gently reoriented toward desire
Dancing reflexes	For flu or similar viruses, or for any aches that permit concentration on other body parts, massage the reflex zones of sexual organs and particular erogenous zones (only when pain is not too dominant).	Amazement at the existence of pleasurable feelings parallel to pain; the possibility of making a conscious decision to concentrate more fully on them

✳ SUGGESTIONS FOR SEXUAL HEALING (CONT'D)

Theme	What to do	Effects on the healing processes
Breast massage	Engage in breast massage (described in Chapter 7)—preferably as a daily habit—at a time when it's easy to indulge yourself (like before going to bed or after showering).	Your menstrual cycle becomes regular (again); lighter blood flow or consciously stopped bleeding; changes in cramps and other symptoms; hormonal changes; firming/enlarging of breasts; cancer prevention; conservation of energy while getting rid of waste matter
Gladdening the heart	Exercise 17 works by transforming sexual energy into deep love for yourself and the world; what follows is a "wide heart," the joy of self-love.	Increasing your heart's energy capacity; gentle expansion and loving self-acceptance; strengthening for the confrontation with illness, injury, and weakness
ESO (extended super orgasm; see Exercise 49) with the laying on of hands	Using the "stop" technique, or the "9-1 rhythm" from Exercise 48, energy is built up in steps and repeatedly guided to the needy spot by the laying on of hands; a small circuit may be created between the yoni and the soles of the feet, which are touching, with legs open.	Noticeable pain reduction, for example, after foot operations; better overall condition
Magical fantasies	Build up energy as described above, but without your hands; just use the power of your imagination.	Changing stomachaches or headaches into comfortable pulsing
Big draw	After taking a deep breath in, hold your breath as long as possible; close all orifices, flex your PC and anus muscles as much as possible. Before breathing out, take one more small breath in through the crown chakra, then relax everything while exhaling. Give yourself over to any feelings, images, movements, and sensations, especially after sexual massages.	Strong, lustful-energetic charging of the entire body, while simultaneously relaxing: floating, flying, happiness, "home movies"

When Sex Can't Work as a
Healing Force

When the main issue is simply surviving, all of the patient's energy is being used to maintain basic vegetative functions, so it is flowing inward and is not available for sensations of arousal on the outer skin. When circulation, heart function, and breathing are severely restricted, feeling, sensing, moving, making sounds, and other expressions of sexual energy are usually affected as well. Also, when pain and weakness dominate, the energy that remains is usually not enough for processes of sexual arousal. If, on the other hand, fear or loneliness dominate, a woman may seek calm contacts that provide security and comfort; at this time, she would rather be held or be able to lean on someone. With infectious diseases, often only limited contact is possible—for example, while using mouth protection.

What Works When Nothing Is
Really Working

* As vitality slowly increases, touching and arousing sexual "favorite places"—cautiously at first, then more passionately—can have an invigorating effect.

* Moderate pain can be lessened through the endorphins produced by passionate petting or sexual fantasies. With good practice, pain can even be changed into pleasurable feelings, since the two arousal processes are closely related.

* With weakness and dizziness, sexual arousal can be purifying, clearing, strengthening, and invigorating.

* Self-love can broaden your perspective and direct it toward your healthy and better loved aspects, while relativizing your perspective on parts that are rejected, sick, painful, deaf, or judged to be ugly.

* Through self-love, you can have the experience of regaining partial body control, which increases your overall physical self-awareness.

* Being accepted and comforted by a loving partner can expedite the healing process, make it easier to accept any lasting problems, and

facilitate (mutual) grieving for that which can no longer be experienced. Loving sexual contact does not necessarily change the perception (yours or that of another) of a partially amputated or recently deformed body part from "ugly" to "beautiful," but a desirous inner perception can change the appearance of your outer image, and loving touches can make it possible to love being touched and to create a tender relationship with yourself and your own shape. This can slowly stimulate the growth of new perceptions of beauty and can even transform an open-backed hospital gown into lingerie.

✳ Being caressed can represent a good counterbalance to the technologized routine of the hospital machinery. It can leave you "wanting more," which can prove invigorating.

✳ Even women who are in comas can be reached through loving caresses and gentle touches, even if they are unable to react.

✳ A lovingly stroked or heartily nibbled woman's body usually has better circulation (which gets rid of more toxins and waste matter), feels healthier and more alive. Pelvic movements can also stimulate digestion, which is usually hindered by a lying-down position.

✳ Breathing and gentle movements, as well as making sounds during sex, can passively massage and stimulate internal organs; energy stored as pain and tension can be released. The energy that is usually used to suppress desire and passion can be set free and transformed from fear- or aggression-tinted energy into desire- and life-giving energy.

How It Works

Sexuality as a healing force works differently from, but just as powerfully as, *self-love* or *partnered love,* as long as its energy level is higher than that of pain or fear. This is particularly true when you have had some practice in redirecting and transforming energy. Of course, it only works when both parties behave sensitively and responsibly toward themselves and each other.

In short, it works

- ✳ with trial and error
- ✳ with playfulness and humor
- ✳ with time and space
- ✳ with devotion and boundaries
- ✳ with practice and frustration
- ✳ with openness to all feelings that can be released
- ✳ with direct communication
- ✳ with respect and dignity
- ✳ with clear boundaries against possible overextension
- ✳ with empathy and responsibility on both sides
- ✳ with the option of still finding something awful about oneself
- ✳ with encounters of the heart
- ✳ with a focus on the here and now (this can't be emphasized enough)

For the healthier partner, this means

- ✳ being in touch with your own handicapped, sick, or weak sides
- ✳ being prepared to allow insecurities to arise and to try out new things
- ✳ being able to see and enjoy the strong, healthy, and even superior sides of the sicker partner
- ✳ broadening your own norms of beauty, mobility, and contact wherever possible
- ✳ not trivializing, glossing over, or forcing a positive perspective onto existing obstacles; instead, allowing yourself to have your own feelings about them
- ✳ making a conscious decision *for* or *against* certain ways of expressing love (to the extent that they are now possible)
- ✳ being cautious about assigning one-sided roles and being aware of their effect on the relationship and the individual

For the more obviously handicapped, sick, or restricted partner, this means

* freeing the other, internally and externally, from the role assignments that can quietly sneak up on her (e.g., the one who always compensates, the satisfier of needs, the prettier one, the adored or envied healthy one, or even the role of a guilty person, the insensitive or ignorant one)

* not waiting in silent expectation, but "explaining" yourself to the other person; cheering her up, and sometimes letting the "pedagogue" speak up with patience or frustration (as in, "I'll tell you what works when it doesn't work the way you're used to")

* taking fear, envy, self-hatred, pain, and sorrow seriously, and learning to express all these feelings

* taking responsibility for your own pleasure, while still seeing the other person and her differences

* being willing to experiment alone, rather than leaving all the seeking and finding to the other person

* except in the context of clearly defined games, not sinking into the mire of chronic power- and powerlessness plays (e.g., the one in the role of the invalid is the "Queen of the shared futon," while the healthier one works her fingers to the bone fulfilling all kinds of necessary and unnecessary tasks)

* actively looking for images and reflections of your own identity as a sexual woman

These suggestions cannot, of course, replace a hospital reform that would truly benefit health; but until then, anyone can start with new pleasure creations in the context of her own everyday life—creations that call into question the idea that sick = apathetic. Anyone can think and talk about what works when nothing is really working.

In short, you can start wherever a little pleasure might be found—even if it's only in talking about it.

Resources

Musical Sound Tapestries and Shots of Energy

As we all know, musical taste varies widely. All the suggestions I have given represent my personal preferences, and almost all the exercises can be done without music, accompanied by the chirping of birds or distant everyday noises. In my experience, however, the right music can act as a channel that, when it has the same wavelength as our energy—the same wavelength as the vibrations promoted by various exercises—can help us improve our own states of vibration. Sometimes music from distant lands helps me get over familiar hindrances that are built into my white, German personality structure. Sometimes nonrhythmic background music helps me find my own—gentle—rhythm or look for a new one. Sometimes strong rhythms and loud sound impulses help energize me and give me courage and strength to do an exercise. Sometimes music helps align the differing vibrations of two or more people; if one of them finds the music distracting, however, it should absolutely be changed or turned off. Sometimes it can also be wonderful to let silence step in after a series of "canned music" and to listen to your inner music.

Some people can sing or hum so beautifully that their spontaneous live music is the best kind to use during the exercises. It's the same when a person can drum or play other rhythm instruments well. I usually prefer that to any CD, no matter how well recorded, since live music, in an exchange between emotions and movements, is much more easily integrated into the process, supporting it in a more organic way.

In general, it is better to forego music than to use music that sounds "wrong" right now! This is especially true because your sense of hearing—

like your sense of smell—is closely connected to your erotic and sexual feelings and to devotion (that is, what is offered to you from the outside). So that this devotion can become pure pleasure, it's a good idea to look for music that suits your tastes, and possibly to introduce it to your partner in a pleasant way.

The following are a few suggestions. The numbers in parentheses refer to the tracks on each CD that I find especially appropriate.

FOR RELAXING AND SWITCHING OVER

Aeoliah: *Chambers of the Heart* (1, 2, 4, 5, 6, 7, 9, 10, 11)

Gomer Edwin Evans: *Music for Beauty* (1, 2)

Arvo Pärt: *Alina* (1, 3, 5)

Gandalf: *From Source to Sea* (1, 3)

Sina Vodjani and Choying Drolma: *Dancing Dakini* (2, 3)

Cesaria Evora: *Al Olympia* (many CDs with similar effects)

Kim Waters and Hans Christian: *Rasa: Devotion*

FOR MEDITATION

Karunesh: *Heart Chakra Meditation*

Toni Scott: *Music for Zen Meditation*

Kundalini Meditation (Osho Active Meditation series)

Chakra Breathing (Osho Active Meditation series)

FOR DANCING

Valdeci Oliveira: *Macarena* (5, 7, 9) [this version is unusual in that it is a female interpretation of pieces usually sung by men.]

Cher: *Believe*

Marla Glen: *This Is Marla Glen* (1, 2, 3, 4, 5, 9) and *Marla la Mamma* (10)

k.d. lang: *All You Can Eat* (1, 2, 8, 10) and *Drag* (2, 6, 7)

Gloria Gaynor: *Greatest Hits* (1, 2, 4, 6, 9, 10, 13, 15)

Madonna: *The Power of Good-Bye* (1, 3, 5, 8, 10, 11)

Virgin Voices 2000 (sampler; 1, 7, 10, 11)

Women's World Voices (sampler; 1, 2, 3, 5, 13, 15)

Khadja Nin: *Sambolera*

FOR SHAKING, STAMPING, RAGING

Mari Boine Persen: *Gula Gula*

Gabrielle Roth: *Ritual* (2, 3, 4, 5, 7) and *Totem* and *La Luna*

James Asher: *Feet in the Soil* (1, 3, 5, 6, 11) and *Raising the Rhythms* (1, 3, 4) and *Tigers of the Raj* (2, 4)

Al Gromer Khan: *Tantra Drums* (1, 2, 4, 5, 6, 7, 8, 9, 10)

Talking Taco Music: *Hearts, Hands, and Hides* (2)

Pili Pili: *Dance Jazz Live 1995* (1, 3, 4, 6, 8)

Masters of Percussion: *Mondobeat* (1, 3, 6, 8, 9, 10)

FOR TENDER AROUSAL

Aeoliah: *The Other Side of the Rainbow* (1, 2, 3, 6, 7, 9,10)

David Darling: *Eight String Religion* (1, 3, 4, 6, 7)

Shantiprem: *Garten der Liebe (Garden of Love)* (1, 2, 4, 6) and *Music for Lovers* (1, 2)

Spiritual Environment: *Tantra* (1, 2)

Raphael and Kutira: *Like an Endless River* (1, 3, 4, 5, 6, 7, 8)

Various: *Mega Sound Effects Vol. 2*

Oliver Serano-Alve: *Vida Para Vida* (1, 2, 3, 4, 5, 6, 8, 12)

Rick Wakeman: *Aspirant Sunset* (3, 6, 8, 10)

Sophia: *Hidden Waters* (2) and *Journey into Love* (1, 2, 3, 5)

Chinmaya Dunster: *Lands of the Dawn*

FOR WILD LUST AND ECSTASY

Kirile Loo: *Lullabies for Husbands* (2, 5, 7, 8, 11, 12)

Ashik: *Gypsy Soul* (1)

Janis Joplin: *Best of Janis Joplin* (2, 11)

Ravi Shankar and Philip Glass: *Passages* (3, 4, 5)

Brian Keane and Omar Faruk: *Fire Dance* (1, 2, 5, 6, 9, 11)

Sirus: *Dancing Butterflies* (1, 2, 3, 5, 6)

Colalaila: *Klezmer Fiesta* (16)

Magic Earth: *Women of Power and Grace* (4, 5, 6, 10)

FOR TRANSFORMATION

Shah: *Kamasutra*

Ailon: *Space Effects*

Sarah Brightman: *La Luna* (2, 3, 10)

Doc Childre: *Heart Zones: Music Proven to Boost Vitality* (1)

FOR RESONATING

Al Gromer Khan: *Mahogany Nights* and *God Perfume*

Frank Lorenzen: *Hands*

FOR HEALING

Gila Antara: *Healing Journey I* (5, 7, 14) and *Healing Journey II* (1, 3, 13)

Carien Wijnen and Friends: *Womyn with Wings* (6, 10, 11, 13, 14, 16)

Desert Wind: *Return to the Goddess* (1, 2, 5, 6, 7, 8, 9, 11, 13) and *Gaia: Earth Goddess* (3, 4, 6, 7, 8, 9, 10, 13) and *Shekhina: Hebrew Goddess* (1, 2, 3, 4, 7, 8, 9, 10, 11)

Cecilia: *Inner Harmony* (1, 4, 8, 9, 10)

Oliver Shanti and Friends: *Listening to the Heart* (1, 2, 3, 5, 6)

Enya: *Shepherd Moons* (2)

On Wings of Song and Robert Gass: *Ancient Mother* (4)

Inspirational Literature

Achterberg, Jeanne, and Barbara Dossey. *Rituals of Healing: Using Imagery for Health and Wellness.* New York: Bantam, 1994.

Allende, Isabel. *Aphrodite: A Memoir of the Senses.* New York: Perennial, 1999.

Anand, Margot. *The Art of Everyday Ecstasy.* New York: Broadway, 1999.

Anand, Margot. *The Art of Sexual Magic: Cultivating Sexual Energy to Transform Your Life.* New York: Tarcher, 1996.

Boston Women's Health Book Collective. *Our Bodies Ourselves for the New Century.* Carmichael, CA: Touchstone Books, 1998.

Bright, Susie. *Full Exposure: Opening Up to Sexual Creativity and Erotic Expression.* San Francisco, CA: HarperSanFrancisco, 2000.

Califia, Pat. *Sapphistry: The Book of Lesbian Sexuality.* Tallahassee, FL: Naiad Press, 1988.

Chia, Mantak, and Maneewan Chia. *Healing Love Through the Tao: Cultivating Female Sexual Energy.* Lodi, NJ: Healing Tao, 1991.

Davis, Laura. *Allies in Healing: When the Person You Love Was Sexually Abused as a Child.* New York: Perennial, 1991.

Dodson, Betty. *Sex for One: The Joy of Selfloving.* New York: Three Rivers Press, 1996.

Ensler, Eve. *The Vagina Monologues: The V-Day Edition.* New York: Villard, 2000.

Hoagland, Sarah Lucia. *Lesbian Ethics: Toward New Values.* Palo Alto, CA: Institute of Lesbian Studies, 1989.

Loulan, JoAnn. *Lesbian Passion: Loving Ourselves and Each Other.* Gardena, CA: Spinsters Ink, 1987.

Muir, Charles, and Caroline Muir. *Tantra: The Art of Conscious Loving.* San Francisco, CA: Mercury House, 1990.

Ogden, Gina. *Women Who Love Sex: An Inquiry into the Expanding Spirit of Women's Erotic Experience.* Cambridge, MA: Womanspirit Press, 1999.

Piontek, Maitreyi D. *Exploring the Hidden Power of Female Sexuality.* Boston, MA: Red Wheel/Weiser, 2001.

Shaw, Miranda. *Passionate Enlightenment: Women in Tantric Buddhism.* Princeton, NJ: Princeton University Press, 1995.

Thadani, Giti. *Sakhiyani: Lesbian Desire in Ancient and Modern India.* London: Cassel, 1996.

Walker, Barbara G. *The Woman's Encyclopedia of Myths and Secrets.* San Francisco, CA: HarperSanFrancisco, 1983.

West, Celeste. *A Lesbian Love Advisor.* San Francisco, CA: Cleis Press, 1989.

Sensual Things, Playthings

Good for Her
(877) 588-0900
www.goodforher.com

Good Vibrations
(800) 289-8423
www.goodvibes.com

Toys in Babeland
(800) 658-9119
www.babeland.com

The Xandria Collection
(800) 242-2823
www.xandria.com

SENSUAL OILS

Blue Moon Herbals
(877) 596-1772
www.bluemoonherbals.com

PaganPath.com

www.paganpath.com/perfume/html

ConsciousChoice

www.consciouschoice.com/herbs/herbs1302.html

AromaWeb

www.aromaweb.com

TANTRA WEBSITES

www.tantra.com

www.tantra-sex.com

www.tantralaboratory.com

www.tao-of-sexuality.com

www.margotanand.com

Index

negative, 114–115; obstacles to, 252; positive, 20; removing inner hindrances for, 217; superior/crazy, 19; ugly, 122

feelings exercise, letting go of: goal, time consideration and, 110; step-by-step process of, 110–111; stumbling blocks dealt with in, 111

female ejaculation: U-spot, G-spot, and, 28–29, 205

female lap-speak exercise, letting being in: goal, time consideration and, 121; step-by-step process in, 121–122; stumbling blocks dealt with in, 122

female sexuality: definition of, 2–3; examples of, 2; male gaze reducing, 15; qualities for liberating, 16–18; self-willed, 19–21; totality of, 19

female vision of joy meditation: giving into light in, 222, 223; goal, time considerations and, 220; light foundation in, 220–222; silence in, 221; song of heart in, 221, 222–223; step-by-step process in, 220–223; stumbling blocks dealt with in, 223

feminine nature, 12

feminists, 12

fever, 248

fire dance, 73

fire drink, 58

fire element: in dancing dragon-woman exercise, 75–76; leaving/releasing, 162; supplication to, 160–161

fire-breathing orgasm exercise, 49, 132, 213, 217; bonding position in, 189; chakras in, 187–189; goal, time considerations and, 187; step-by-step process in, 187–188; stumbling blocks dealt with in, 188–189

firewater, 211

flattening massage, letting yourself be comfortable in: goal, time considerations and, 108; step-by-step process in, 108–110; stumbling blocks dealt with in, 110

flute. *See* inner-flute exercise, opening

food, 124, 164, 167

full-moon meditation, 223; goal, time considerations and, 224; step-by-step process in, 224–226; stumbling blocks dealt with in, 226

G

generosity, 16–17

gentlest temptation, 248

giant-woman orgasm, 40

gladdening-the-heart exercise, 49, 102; goal, time considerations and, 103; healing aspect of, 249; sexual self-love with, 49, 102–104; step-by-step process of, 103–104; stumbling blocks dealt with in, 104

gladdening-the-heart exercise, in three-part harmony, 149; goal, time considerations and, 150; step-by-step process in, 150–151; stumbling blocks dealt with in, 151–152

goddesses, 13, 159; lessening of, 15

goddess-point, ringing, 205

good-bye to young girl's self-limitation exercise, saying: goal of, 77; step-by-step process in, 77–78; stumbling blocks dealt with in, 78

Gräfenberg, Mr., 28

groaning yoni and laughing belly exercise, 117; goal, time consideration and, 118; step-by-step process of, 118–119; stumbling blocks dealt with in, 119

G-spot, 36, 194, 201; female ejaculation and, 28–29, 205; magic "mussel" massage of, 204–205, 206; orgasm's edge with, 206; physical aspect of, 28; for stimulating orgasm, 210–211

guilt, 245–246

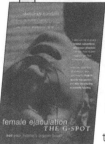
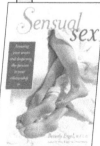